"This is a fascinating book filled ' from a lifetime of treating thousands of pat...

Wayne Grudem, Research Professor of Theology and Biblical Studies, Phoenix Seminary

"This book is full of strategies for life's second half. Its advice is practical and priceless."

David Stevens, CEO, Christian Medical and Dental Associations

"Dr. Dunlop speaks from a wealth of personal experience as a beloved physician to countless older people, watching them live and die well—and poorly. A lifelong and careful study of the Bible has given him an invaluable perspective on how to 'run with endurance the race that is set before us.' We long to keep up, and even to excel, but how? If you want a wealth of biblically sound and immensely practical strategies for staying well, you've come to the right place. This book is a treasure!"

John F. Kilner, PhD, Professor of Bioethics and Contemporary Culture and Forman Chair of Ethics and Theology, Trinity Evangelical Divinity School

"In today's busy medical practice, doctors rarely have the time to sit down and share all the advice needed to keep patients well. Here, in one volume, Dr. Dunlop has collected everything I wish I had time to teach my patients."

Harry Kraus, MD, board-certified surgeon; best-selling author, *Lip Reading* and *Domesticated Jesus*

"A deep reading of the book reveals many pearls that the disciplined and attentive physician John Dunlop has uncovered over the years of taking care of elderly patients and observing their lives, as well as his own. This book will challenge your thinking and your doing."

D. Joy Riley, MD, MA, Executive Director, The Tennessee Center for Bioethics and Culture; author, *Outside the Womb* and *Christian Bioethics*

"The desire to be well and the reading of Dunlop's book run on parallel tracks. Heading into their senior years, readers who don't have the time or the expertise to thoroughly research the issues facing them—issues about which they must make decisions before it's too late—will find this a well-organized and right-sized aid. I found his brief section on dementia and memory loss especially helpful."

Sam Crabtree, Executive Pastor, Bethlehem Baptist Church, Minneapolis, Minnesota; author, *Practicing Affirmation*

"Refreshingly holistic and consistent with the biblical concept of *shalom*, rather than the material-spiritual dualism so common in contemporary Christian thought, Dunlop addresses not only physical and mental wellness but also social, financial, spiritual, and emotional wellness. I'm already applying some of its lessons and pray many others will use it to help them improve the extent to which they live well for the glory of God!"

Sharon A. Falkenheimer, MA, MD, MPH, Associate Fellow of the Center for Bioethics and Human Dignity, Trinity International University; Clinical Assistant Professor in the Department of Preventative Medicine and Community Health, The University of Texas at Galveston

"Drawing from decades as a caring and compassionate physician, Dr. Dunlop shares insights and strategies about life choices that result in successful aging. He provides actual patient vignettes, which clearly illustrate the biblical basis for wellness and wholeness that go beyond just physical health. He challenges readers to prayerful self-examination that can lead to sound and lasting change. His tone is pastoral and personal, as if he were sitting alongside the reader and gently counseling. The chapters are sprinkled with humor and include many good references for those who want deeper understanding. This book encompasses all we need to hear from someone who is wise and godly."

Clydette Powell, MD, MPH, FAAP, Associate Professor of Pediatrics, Division of Child Neurology, The George Washington University School of Medicine and Health

Wellness
FOR THE
Glory
OF
God

LIVING WELL AFTER 40
WITH JOY AND CONTENTMENT IN ALL OF LIFE

John Dunlop, MD

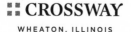

CROSSWAY

WHEATON, ILLINOIS

Wellness for the Glory of God: Living Well after 40 with Joy and Contentment in All of Life

Copyright © 2014 by John Dunlop, MD

Published by Crossway
           1300 Crescent Street
           Wheaton, Illinois 60187

Material by Jonathan Edwards is taken from *God's Passion for His Glory* by John Piper, ©1998. Used by permission of Crossway, a publishing ministry of Good News Publishers, Wheaton, IL 60187, www.crossway.org.

Cover design: Faceout Studio

First printing 2014

Printed in the United States of America

Unless otherwise indicated, Scripture quotations are from the ESV® Bible (*The Holy Bible, English Standard Version®*), copyright © 2001 by Crossway. 2011 Text Edition. Used by permission. All rights reserved.

Scripture quotations marked NIV are taken from *The Holy Bible, New International Version®*, NIV®. Copyright © 1973, 1978, 1984 by Biblica, Inc.™ Used by permission. All rights reserved worldwide.

Trade paperback ISBN: 978-1-4335-3812-4
ePub ISBN: 978-1-4335-3815-5
PDF ISBN: 978-1-4335-3813-1
Mobipocket ISBN: 978-1-4335-3814-8

Library of Congress Cataloging-in-Publication Data

Dunlop, John, 1947–
    Wellness for the glory of God : living well after 40 with joy and contentment in all of life / John Dunlop, MD.
        pages cm
    Includes bibliographical references and index.
    ISBN 978-1-4335-3812-4 (tp)
    1. Middle-aged persons—Religious life. 2. Well-being—Religious aspects—Christianity. 3. Quality of life—Religious aspects—Christianity. I. Title.
BV4579.5.D86   2014
248.8'5—dc23   2014006666

Crossway is a publishing ministry of Good News Publishers.

VP   24 23 22 21 20 19 18 17 16 15 14
15 14 13 12 11 10 9 8 7 6 5 4 3 2 1

To my patients and
coworkers in Zion who
have been my friends
and teachers

Contents

Introduction

Henry came into the examining room huffing and puffing, using his walker to get down the hall. I shook his hand and asked, "How is it going my friend?" Smiling, he gave me a strong handshake and said, "Praise the Lord, I'm well, thank you!" As pleased as I was to hear his response, it caught me just a bit off-guard. I was sixty-five; he was ninety-five! I found myself wanting to be like that thirty years from now. Then all kinds of questions began to pop into my mind:

- What does it mean to be well at ninety-five: short of breath and using our walkers?

- Will I be able to say I'm well if I am still on earth at that age?

- What can I do now to increase the chance of being well in thirty years?

Having practiced medicine, with a special emphasis on geriatrics, since 1976, I have seen a lot of folks move through their older years. A significant percentage of my patients are Christians. I am impressed at how different the later days of life can generally be for those who embrace faith in Christ compared to those who do not. However, there are no universal rules for growing old successfully. Some, Christian or not, seem to thrive and continue to grow as life's end approaches; others slowly fade away without joy or a sense of completion. I am fully aware that much of what makes the difference between the two is outside of man's control. Yet I am equally convinced that some is within man's control. I often tell my patients that the difference between ninety-five-year-olds in the nursing home and those on the golf course is the choices they made in their sixties. That is what this book is about.

What strategies can we who are getting older adopt that will maximize our chances to endure the challenges of our later days and continue to be well? The essence of this book is expressed in the title. Wellness depends on living with a purpose that goes beyond the here and now. Over and over I have seen that one way in which Christians can stay well in their twilight years is to keep their focus on God, his greatness, and his glory.

Born in 1947, I am well into my second half of life. That makes me a Baby Boomer, a member of the generation that arrived between 1946 and 1964. I suspect that many of you are Boomers too. As Boomers, we are close to retirement and confronting the fact that our lives are more than half over. I remind my patients that getting older means two things: first, we are not old yet, but we're getting there; and, second, we're not dead yet! They say, "Old dogs can't learn new tricks." That may be true, but remember that we are still just *getting* older, so there is time to change. If we are going to age successfully, we need to think carefully about what we want to be like when we are old, take stock of where we are now, and develop strategies to move us from here to there. We need to consider all domains of wellness to get a complete picture.

In this book we will examine physical, mental, social, financial, spiritual, and emotional wellness. As you read, I will share stories of people who are quite old and doing well. Many of these are real people, though their names are altered. In some cases I have combined several stories to make a point; others are purely fictitious. These examples allow us to see what being well in the later years can look like and what strategies we can implement now to increase our chance of continuing to be well.

There is great value in our older years. They are an important part of our lives. We dare not look at these years as putting in time till God calls us home. That unfortunately may be the default of our culture, but as Christians we must not allow that thinking. The changes we experience as we age are nothing to be embarrassed about. No! Proverbs 16:31 tells us, "Gray hair is a crown of glory." The effects of aging are clear evidence of God's blessing. Even our increasing dependence on others need not deny our intrinsic value. We must see our value as rooted in the fact that we are made in God's image and redeemed by Christ, not in what we can accomplish. For way too long, we have faced getting older with some degree of apprehension and dread. Now it is time to see a more positive picture. Statistically, our generation is likely to live longer than any generation since ancient times. God does not make mistakes. He is allowing this longevity for a definite reason. We need to find the purpose he has for our older years and pursue it with vigor.

I have a lot to share with you and want to propose a number of strategies for you to think over. I am writing as if you were one of my patients, and we are chatting together at my office. I love such conversations, but often there is just too much to talk about in the limited time we have together, so I have put these suggestions in writing for you.

This book is not intended to be a comfortable read. Even while writing I have been challenged to make some changes in my own life. I pray that these thoughts will challenge you as well. As I share my strategies with you, stop, think, and pray that God will show you how you are doing in that area. When you think of changes you need to make, turn to the back of the book where you can write down specific steps to take. Make yourself accountable and write down dates by which you feel you can make the change. Don't limit yourself to the suggestions I make. Allow God, by his Spirit, to speak to you and prompt you about other necessary changes.

You will note that this book is written specifically for and about Christians. If you are truly a Christian, I trust you will find these chapters encouraging as you look forward to further years knowing God on this earth and, even more, to spending your eternity with God in heaven. Some of you have lived a "good Christian life" but find that the way of life I am talking about here goes far beyond your experience. I would urge you to find a godly pastor or friend and talk over your reactions.

Perhaps you do not view yourself as Christian. Please read on, for many of the strategies I present are equally valid for you, and perhaps you will see that the Christian faith makes sense and that there is a lot of wisdom in the Scriptures I quote. Several friends suggested I write a book without a strong spiritual emphasis, yet I chose not to do so since a strong faith is critical to successful aging. I felt it imperative to write within a spiritual, and in this case, Christian, context.

A book like this never comes out of a vacuum. As you will see, I ground many of my strategies in the Bible. I trust you will see the quotes as illustrative of what the Bible teaches as a whole and not just as isolated passages intended to prove my point. I had the privilege of growing up under the tutelage of wise and godly parents who had a lasting impact on my life. My years of medical practice allowed me to observe how many patients stayed well to the glory of God, and I learned much from them. Though it seems ironic to say, many were quite well when they died.

It is impossible to give individual credit to many of the dear friends whose impact I have felt, but, without a doubt, God has greatly used them to shape the thinking expressed in this volume. I owe a significant debt to each. One who deserves specific mention is Dr. Charles (Chick) Sell, who has spent countless hours helping me put "doctor talk" into writing that you can understand. I am also indebted to my wife, Dorothy, my two sons, Jamie and Rob, and friends such as Rose Bowen, Nate and Sharon Hale, and Donna Crum, who have read the manuscript and offered wise counsel. Finally, I want to thank Lydia Brownback of Crossway for her careful editing.

Before we get into our first chapter, take a moment and reflect on the challenge we have in the Scriptures:

Do you not know that in a race all the runners run, but only one receives the prize? So run that you may obtain it. Every athlete exercises self-control in all things. They do it to receive a perishable wreath, but we an imperishable. So I do not run aimlessly; I do not box as one beating the air. But I discipline my body and keep it under control, lest after preaching to others I myself should be disqualified. (1 Cor. 9:24–27)

Therefore, since we are surrounded by so great a cloud of witnesses, let us also lay aside every weight, and sin which clings so closely, and let us run with endurance the race that is set before us. (Heb. 12:1)

Life really is like a race, and, as any runner knows, the end of the race is the hardest. Think for just a moment about who is there at the finish line. It is Jesus, the one who died for us. As soon as we cross the finish line, we will be invited to "enter into the joy of [our] master" (Matt. 25:21). But even as we run, we are surrounded by a great cloud of witnesses who have already finished their race. The church triumphant is cheering us on. I can almost hear them shouting, "Stay well! Run hard! It won't be too much farther." My prayer is that you will find in this book useful strategies to stay well to the end, so that God will be glorified in your life and in the lives of those who are watching you.

Prayer

Father,
I am attracted to the concept of staying well to the glory of God. Speak to me through your Word by your Spirit as I read and help me examine my life to know what changes I need to make. Renew my passion for you. Help me to offer the remaining days I have on earth as a sacrifice to you. Give me wisdom; show me the way. Grant me strength to run hard to the end and allow me to experience joy along the way. May it all be to your glory.
Amen

1

What Is Wellness?

Most of us who would meet Joan would say that she is anything but well. At sixty-eight she has been in a wheelchair for twenty-six years, the victim of aggressive multiple sclerosis. She lives by herself, her husband having divorced her many years ago; but she is closely attended by her three children and a myriad of friends from her church. She gets by with equipment that allows her to move around in the apartment, prepare simple meals, and do some basic housework. Still, she suffers frequently from disabling fatigue. In addition to requiring eight hours of sleep at night, she has to rest in bed for four hours during the day. The remainder of her time is spent reading and keeping up an e-mail correspondence with people all over the world, for whom she maintains an active prayer ministry. Four to five times a week, various friends stop by for a cup of tea. It's amazing how many respond in the same way: "You know, I always plan to stop by and cheer up Joan, but the fact is, she invariably cheers me up. She doesn't deny her problems but chooses not to dwell on them. Her love for God is absolutely contagious."

Jim is seventy-two. An avid runner, he tries to log at least twenty miles a week. He keeps up a good pace and can do a seven-minute mile if he pushes himself. He spends at least three hours at the gym four days a week, and the days he is not there, he is out taking long walks by himself. But that's just the problem—he's always by himself. Jim can greet the regulars at the gym by name but has no close friends. He is acutely aware that if he didn't show up, no one would miss him. His ex-wife is happily remarried, and his children have had nothing to do with him since he left the family twenty-five years ago.

Mary, at eighty-eight, is moderately demented. She lives with her daughter, Beth, and is able to help out with the dishes and light housework early in the day but typically gets more confused and agitated during the evening hours. Beth has found that when confusion occurs, she can play some Christian music from thirty years ago. Mary has always loved these hymns, and she relaxes as she sings along with the old songs.

Now, allow me to ask the key question: Which one of these three is truly well? When asked, "How are you?" which one could honestly smile and say, "I'm well, thank you." Would it be Joan with her MS; Jim, the seven-minute miler; or Mary with her dementia?

What is wellness, anyway? At first blush most of us would answer in terms of our physical health. Have you heard about the Turbaned Tornado? This is Fauja Singh, who completed the Toronto Marathon when he was one hundred years old. You may say, "Wow, he was certainly well." I agree that you don't run a marathon when you are sick. But is physical health all there is to wellness? If wellness requires us to complete a marathon at one hundred, most of us won't make it. Thankfully, wellness is much more than physical health and freedom from distressing symptoms. Wellness involves the whole of our being, which includes six distinct areas: physical, mental, social, financial, spiritual, and emotional. These areas of wellness are not independent but are all interrelated. Each area contributes to the well-being of each of the others. At the same time, struggles in one area may detract from wellness in each of the others.

In dealing with aging patients, I have observed that having a sense of wellness sometimes results from placing sufficient value on at least one area of life where things are going well in order to trump areas where things could improve. Over the years I have heard many say, "If I can just stay healthy, that is all I want." Yet I have seen many in great health who could not be called "well." Jim, who at seventy-two is running twenty miles a week, is a case in point. His physical well-being is not enough to compensate for the other areas where he is lacking.

Furthermore, if we are going to choose one area in which to ground our sense of wellness, we want to make sure it will last throughout our lives. That may be the problem with both our physical and mental health—they may begin to run down. So it is with most of the other domains of wellness. Emotionally upbeat people may experience many losses that erode their optimism. Many experience their financial security disappearing when the economy takes a downturn. Those who are counting on family and friends may experience severe disappointments. But there is one area of wellness that need not fail—our relationship with God.

I will never forget dear Eddie, who, when I told her she had only a matter of weeks till her colon cancer would take her life, looked at me incredulous that I thought I was giving her bad news. Her response was, "Well, you don't get to heaven by being healthy, do you?" Even facing death, Eddie felt well because she placed more value on spiritual realities than on physical. Maintaining spiritual wellness can be of great benefit in this life, and it is the only area of wellness that we will continue to enjoy throughout eternity. Paul wrote:

> We do not lose heart. Though our outer nature is wasting away, our inner nature is being renewed day by day. For this light momentary affliction is preparing for us an eternal weight of glory beyond all comparison, as we look not to the things that are seen but to the things that are unseen. For the things that are seen are transient, but the things that are unseen are eternal. (2 Cor. 4:16–18)

Paul would have been one of those who could answer, "I'm well, thank you," even as his outer nature wasted away.

Late in his life John wrote his third epistle. It was addressed to his beloved friend Gaius, and in it John said, "I pray that all may go well with you and that you may be in good health, as it goes well with your soul" (3 John 2). John equated good health not with the state of Gaius's body but with the state of his soul. A healthy spirit can help compensate for difficulties faced in each of the other areas. But that must not be our only focus, for maintaining wellness in the other five areas contributes to our spiritual wellness. Keeping physically and mentally healthy allows us to get out and serve others while continuing to grow in our understanding of God. Social relationships are so often key to spiritual wellness. Learning to trust God for our finances and maintaining a positive outlook will similarly contribute to our spiritual health. The bottom line is that our top priority—spiritual wellness—is best nurtured in the context of staying well in as many of the other areas as possible.

Staying Well Requires Planning

Yogi Berra said, "If you don't know where you are going, you might wind up someplace else."[1] That applies to wellness. We need to carefully define our goals, choose the wisest strategies to accomplish them, and discipline ourselves to implement those strategies if we are going to maximize the chance that we can be well in as many spheres as possible.

Even with that, the overachievers among us will have to recognize that it is far-fetched to think that we will have true wellness in all six areas of life at the same time. God in his sovereignty may overrule and have reasons for us to go through seasons where we are not well. The difficulties we face may be the result of living in a world affected by sin, or they may be the natural consequences of bad choices we have made.

Let's face it: most of us are not going to die while we are physically healthy or free from difficulties. Paul and Barnabas taught the new believers in Asia Minor "that through many tribulations we must enter the kingdom of God" (Acts 14:22). Paul himself experienced "many tribulations" including being stoned and left for dead, receiving the notorious thirty-nine lashes five times, and being shipwrecked three times while being left afloat at sea for a day and a night! Recall that he referred to these as "light momentary affliction." Why? It is because such difficulties are "preparing for us an eternal weight of glory beyond all comparison" (2 Cor. 4:17). Paul experienced wellness not through the absence of problems but through his abiding confidence that God was in control and that in eternity he would see God's ultimate purpose.

Even while we realize that in some areas of our lives, God may overrule our best intentions—and we want him to accomplish his purposes for us—we should still set wellness as our goal. To do that, we must first understand what wellness is, think carefully through each sphere of life, and identify strategies to maintain wellness.

Wellness Defined

I define wellness as *that blessed state of experiencing all spheres of life functioning in harmony with God's ordained purpose.* Let us unpack that statement.

> *blessed* . . . is a word frequently used in both Old and New Testaments. It speaks of a state of good fortune, being well off and happy. True blessing is a gift from God, not something we earn. We have some responsibility to create an environment where he can work, but fundamentally it is God who graciously blesses us. Even the things we do to pursue wellness are possible because he gives us the wisdom, motivation, and ability.

21

state of experiencing . . . emphasizes that wellness is not just an objective fact but a subjective experience. It allows us to say not only, "I am well," but also, "I feel well."

all spheres of life . . . indicates that wellness involves the whole person. It includes all six areas we are considering.

functioning . . . implies that wellness is not only a state of being but is also what we do.

in harmony with . . . suggests the deep, satisfying peace that comes from sharing together and being united with something that is much bigger than ourselves.

God's ordained purpose. To be well we need a purpose that gives meaning and significance to our lives today and will continue to do so until the day we die. What better purpose could we have than being part of God's *eternal* purpose and allowing him to dictate how every part of our lives will contribute to his overall plan? Right from the start we need to appreciate that being in harmony with God's ordained purpose does not mean everything will be sunshine and roses, since his plan will include difficulties. When I struggle in life, I often quote from one of my favorite psalms: "One thing God has spoken, two things have I heard: that you, O God, are strong, and that you, O LORD, are loving" (Ps. 62:11–12 NIV). If I affirm that God is able to do what he wants (he is strong) and that he is loving, I can joyfully conclude that everything that happens is under his control and will result in what he knows is best. This is the gist of what Paul writes: "We know that for those who love God all things work together for good, for those who are called according to his purpose" (Rom. 8:28). Once I am in harmony with God's purpose, I can be well, regardless of my circumstances. I can know I am in the right spot, and I can rest comfortably.

To take this a step further, we need to understand how wellness necessitates being in harmony with God and then what his purposes are.

Shalom and Shema

The ancient Hebrews contribute to our understanding of harmony and thereby wellness by their use of the word *shalom*. Whereas *shalom* is loosely translated "peace," the true meaning is far more extensive; at root it means "totality."[2] It is the sense of wholeness we have when every part of our lives is in a profound harmony and unity within ourselves, with those around us, and with God. Wellness requires *shalom*.

Where do we find the integrating principle that brings every area of our lives together? Once again, the ancient Jews had the correct answer. The famous Shema of Israel says, "Hear, O Israel: The LORD our God, the LORD is one. You shall love the LORD your God with all your heart and with all your soul and with all your might" (Deut. 6:4–5). We are to be a people of one God. This must be more than something we recite, for we need to have him as our single focus and see all other areas of life from his perspective. We are to love him with all our heart, soul, and might. The word "might" is interesting, for it means nothing less than our everything. Love is not onerous, nor is it something we try to avoid. Who does not want to experience love? Yet God, the all-powerful sovereign of the universe, desires to have a loving relationship with us. That does not mean I cannot love other people and many of the good things God has given me to enjoy in this life, but it does mean that my ultimate purpose is to love him, and loving others becomes a means to that end.

Love for God is well illustrated in the Scriptures:

O God, you are my God; earnestly I seek you;
    my soul thirsts for you;
my flesh faints for you,
    as in a dry and weary land where there is no water.
So I have looked upon you in the sanctuary,
    beholding your power and glory.

> Because your steadfast love is better than life,
>> my lips will praise you. (Ps. 63:1–3)

It is not just that we are to love God; we have spoken of the loving *relationship* we have with God. Relationships are, after all, two-way streets. We are not responsible to come up with a love for God by ourselves; rather, our love for him and for others is the natural response of his love for us.

> Christ may dwell in your hearts through faith—that you, being rooted and grounded in love, may have strength to comprehend with all the saints what is the breadth and length and height and depth, and to know the love of Christ that surpasses knowledge, that you may be filled with all the fullness of God. (Eph. 3:17–19)

> We love because he first loved us. (1 John 4:19)

We learn to love God with all of our being and then find in him our fulfillment and greatest joy. In God we find what we need to be satisfied. We experience *shalom* through Shema and can pursue wellness.

I have been blessed to know many who have found great peace in pursuing God's purpose with all of their being. I think of Carolyn, who at eighty-seven is living with her severely demented husband. At this stage of life, he is her total preoccupation, and this is her way of loving God. I have never heard her complain, because she has a deep sense that she is exactly where the Lord wants her at this time. She is content to be in God's will. That does not make her life easy, but it does allow her to experience *shalom*.

And there are Will and Sandy. Will retired at seventy as a carpenter and Sandy several years earlier from her job in a school cafeteria. They sold their house and bought a motor home. Now they spend at least six months a year visiting Christian camps where Will does repair work and Sandy works in the kitchen. Whenever I see them, they can't stop raving about how happy they are. They know this is where they belong and are experiencing God's *shalom*.

Then there is Jack, who was widowed after sixty-four years of marriage. He gets lonely at times, and although very limited by arthritis he gets out to two different Bible studies each week, and once a week he goes to visit the people from his church who are in a nursing home. I have frequently asked Jack how he is doing, and his typical response is, "Well, it's tough, but I'm getting by."

It may not seem as though any of these individuals are doing life-shaking things, but they are fulfilling God's purpose and are experiencing wellness. Yet while loving God and loving other people are wonderful and may lead to our ultimate purpose, they are not that ultimate purpose in themselves. To attain that ultimate goal we must go one level deeper.

Pursue God's Glory[3]

Our overriding purpose in life should be to glorify God. There are many ways in which God can be glorified. For example, God is glorified when we worship, praise, value, honor, thank, enjoy, or even emulate him. To understand how God is glorified, we need first to realize that glorifying him is not something we initiate. It is not as if we are light bulbs that send forth our own light to reveal God's goodness. Rather, we are mirrors that reflect the goodness we have received from him.

We must also understand that we can bring God glory in three distinct ways. First, he is glorified in our spirit as we find greater joy and fulfillment in him. Second, others may give him glory as a result of something we do for them that reflects God's love and goodness. Third, God is glorified in his own being through our worship as we declare how much we treasure him. The apostle Paul speaks of Christians as being "the aroma of Christ to God" (2 Cor. 2:15). It is difficult to understand fully, but in some way we remind God of the sacrifice of his beloved son, Jesus, who allowed us to come to God.

The Scriptures clearly state that God's purpose for creation is his glory. Through Isaiah God refers to "everyone who is called by my name, whom I created for my glory" (43:7). God's glory is not only the purpose of creation but also the reason God allows us to put our hope for eternal life in Jesus's death for us: "We who were the first to hope in Christ might be to the praise of his glory" (Eph. 1:12). When we trust Christ, we are saved from the punishment we deserve for our sin and are made a part of Christ's body on earth, the church. The ultimate purpose of the church is that God be glorified. "To him be glory in the church and in Christ Jesus throughout all generations, forever and ever. Amen" (Eph. 3:21). Paul could not have put it more succinctly: "For from him and through him and to him are all things. To him be glory forever. Amen" (Rom. 11:36). God's desire to evidence his glory is the ultimate reason for creation (from him); it is the means by which all things are sustained (through him) and the final climax to which it is headed (to him).

Some say that God must be terribly self-absorbed to be so concerned about his own glory. Admittedly, from our finite and sinful human perspective that does seem true. If we respond that way, we need to remember that one of the characteristics of a good person is to love what is truly good. Then, when we remember that God alone is the essence of goodness, it should be expected that he will desire us to enjoy and glorify his goodness.

What Are the Results of Living with a Passion for God's Glory?

It will free us from worry and anxiety. Once our passion is for the glory of God, we will be less concerned about ourselves and, consequently, not experience as much anxiety, worry, or fear.

We will function out of a sense of fullness, not emptiness. When we are focused on God and his glory more than on ourselves, we are able to find our fullness in him. We overflow in giving to others rather than just looking for affirmation from them.

It will energize us and ignite us with passion. A passion for God's glory should encourage and ignite within us a longing to serve God to the utmost of our abilities. We do not want to be unrealistic here, since, as the years go by, we may be more limited in our abilities. Still, we can give everything we have.

We will fulfill our eternal purpose, find our niche, feel at home, and be content. It is never comfortable to do something that we feel neither called nor equipped to do. That will never be the case when we are living for God and his glory.

We will do things with eternal impact. We were made for something bigger than this world. As we live for God's glory, the things we do may have lasting eternal impact and value.

Shema and shalom. When our love for God and passion for his glory (Shema) become the unifying focus of our lives, we will experience *shalom*.

We will continue to pursue God for all eternity. Wellness does not have to wait until we experience God in his fullness. Experiencing God's fullness can never happen in this life, and the reality is that it cannot even be attained in eternity. But that is good, for I am not really well if I sit back and relax, thinking that I have arrived. No, I am only well when I am moving forward, when I am growing. This is particularly true of my relationship to God. The riches of God are infinite, and it will take an infinite amount of time (eternity) to plumb the depths of our infinite God. We will continue to grow in our understanding of God throughout eternity, and in the process of growing we will experience true wellness.

What Is the Next Step?

If we are to aim for the unity in our lives that allows for true wellness, we need to consider each part of our lives and examine how it fits into this big picture. We need to consider our physical, mental, social, financial, spiritual, and emotional states and determine how they could better allow us to live to the glory of God. Next, we consider physical wellness.

Questions for Reflection and Discussion

Before progressing to the rest of this book, take a moment for personal evaluation:

Fill in the blanks: God's chief purpose for my life is that I will G _ _ _ _ _ _ H _ _. This is often accomplished by my L _ _ _ for him and for O _ _ _ _ _.

Define *shalom*.

_____

_____

_____

What is the unifying purpose of your life?

_____

_____

_____

Pretend you are a teacher and give yourself a grade for how well you are doing in each of the areas below. Mark it A, B, C, D, or F. Then jot down any changes you already know you need to make.

Area	Grade	Changes I need
Physical	_____	_____
Mental	_____	_____
Social	_____	_____
Financial	_____	_____
Spiritual	_____	_____
Emotional	_____	_____

Prayer

Father,

It is likely that you will grant me more years to live on this earth before you call me home. I want them to bring you glory. I pray that you will guide me as I read through these chapters. Capture my affections and allow me to love you more. Allow me to experience *shalom* as I learn to have greater focus so that all areas of my life work together and count for you. I pray this, knowing that what is best for me is that you will be glorified.

Amen

2

Physical Wellness

A HEALTHY LIFESTYLE

At fifty-five, Pete was feeling great. His youngest had just left for college, and he and his wife were starting to enjoy their empty nest. With six weeks of paid time off from his stressful job, he and Jennie were planning to make the most of them. Having always wanted to travel abroad, they now had their chance. That is, until Pete came in for a physical. He had not been exercising and was about fifty pounds overweight. He had started to notice some discomfort in his chest after climbing more than two flights of stairs. In his routine exam he had some blood in his stool. His lab work revealed iron deficiency anemia, and his electrocardiogram showed some worrisome changes. It was off to the cardiac stress lab, where Pete's nuclear study revealed that a significant part of his heart muscle was not getting enough oxygen. After another test showed that several of his arteries were clogged, he underwent a four-vessel bypass operation. As he was recovering from that, he had a colonoscopy, which showed a premalignant polyp that had been oozing blood. It was removed without surgery.

Take Good Care of Your Body

Suffice it to say that Pete and Jennie had a major wake-up call. Their diet changed dramatically. No longer were there steaks on the grill every weekend. Breakfast was not sausage and eggs. Fast food became a thing of the past. Up at six o'clock every morning, they did a two-mile walk before Pete left for work. Over the next year Pete lost those extra fifty pounds and couldn't believe how much better he felt. At the time of his next annual physical he was a totally different person. I remember seeing him beaming as he pointed to the new holes in his belt. What a transformation Pete had made. I was waiting for his next words, and, sure enough, they came as I would have predicted: "John, why didn't I make these changes years ago?"

Physical wellness is rarely related to a single factor. Some of its roots are beyond our control, perhaps hidden in our genes. Some are simply the results of living in a world where bad things happen. Yet many are the predictable consequences of the poor choices we make. In this chapter, it is these preventable things that I want to focus on.

It intrigues me that a healthy lifestyle is rarely rocket science, and most of us have a general idea of how to maintain one. Rarely is the problem not knowing what to do. More often, it is not having the will to do it or, even more frequently, the discipline to stick to it. I am never certain how to motivate my patients to change their lifestyle. Often it takes a distressful wake-up call such as the one that shocked Pete, but sometimes even that is not enough. Since education can help us understand what to do, I will try to offer you some practical ways to avoid such a crisis and stay as healthy as possible. Education can also allow us to understand some of the consequences of not doing what we should. But for Christians, I believe there is a much stronger reason to do what we can to stay healthy. Allow me to set the background from Scripture.

In Old Testament times God took up residence in the tabernacle, where the cloud of his glory was present above the ark of the covenant. He gave very explicit instructions for the care of the tabernacle. Later the ark was moved into Solomon's temple, where God's presence remained until the prophet Ezekiel saw God's glory leave. God did not take up a specific residence on earth until the time of Christ's incarnation. Then he was present in the person of

Jesus. When Christ ascended back to the Father, the presence of God returned to man when his Spirit came at Pentecost to indwell believers. Now he lives in us. "Or do you not know that your body is a temple of the Holy Spirit within you, whom you have from God? You are not your own, for you were bought with a price. So glorify God in your body" (1 Cor. 6:19–20). We must be careful how we use the phrase "my body," for in truth it belongs to God. He has entrusted its care to us. He expects us to keep it healthy, clean, and fit for his residence and use. There can be no pulling punches here—that is a very strong reason to pursue physical wellness. Paul wrote, "I discipline my body and keep it under control" (1 Cor. 9:27). That is exactly what we need to do. Therefore, our first strategy toward wellness for *the glory of God* is to adopt a healthy lifestyle.

Guidelines for Healthy Living

So how do we go about taking good care of our bodies? Good physical health results from following some basic guidelines.

Manage Your Weight

Weight is a major health problem for many and has now reached epidemic proportions. Obesity can lead to diabetes, arthritis, premature heart disease, stroke, and many forms of cancer. In short, it compromises both the length of our lives and our ability to keep active. I am not sure we have a clear scientific understanding

> **STRATEGY**
> Take good care of your body, for it is the temple of the Holy Spirit.

of all the root causes of obesity. I suspect that there may be as many causes of obesity as there are people who suffer from it. For some, it is financial: foods that lead to obesity are cheaper. For others, it is a community problem: there are no safe places to exercise. For others, the causes are hormonal or genetic. There is good evidence that inadequate sleep leads to obesity. In certain cases, obesity comes from eating behavior passed on through family traditions. In other cases, people eat too much in response to stress or depression. Obesity can even be a spiritual problem, when we seek in food the satisfaction that we can find only in the Lord. While the causes are multiple, the treatment always boils down to first identifying and dealing with the root cause and then figuring out some way to burn more calories than we consume. It may be easier when we recognize that some calories are more satisfying than others. There is no question that a one-hundred-calorie serving of broccoli is much more filling than one hundred calories of butter. I encourage my patients to use a calorie-restricted diet and to exercise to lose weight and keep it off. Although necessary, I admit it is not easy.

Get Plenty of Exercise

I have on my desk a card that quotes Robert Butler, a specialist in geriatric medicine. It simply says, "If exercise could be packed in a pill, it would be the single most widely prescribed and beneficial medicine in the nation." Dr. Butler highlights two things. First, exercise is of inestimable value; and, second, we prefer to take pills for everything that ails us because they are the easier solution. Fundamentally we are lazy.

But how much exercise is enough? For many of us, the answer seems to be "Just a little bit more." Yet as little as twenty minutes a day or 150 minutes a week will help maintain good health, and twice that will help you lose weight. Our exercise should take four forms: aerobic to keep us moving and keep our hearts healthy; anaerobic for muscle toning; stretching; and balance training. We should keep in mind that none of these needs to be a formal gym workout. The key is to keep physically active while doing something we enjoy. It is also important to choose activities that we can do year-round. As we age, our approach to exercise will inevitably change; but we should realize that poor health is rarely a reason not to keep physically active.

When it comes to aerobic exercise, I have traditionally gone beyond the minimum and recommend three hours a week, or thirty minutes six days a week. A brisk thirty-minute walk accomplishes that, but there are many other options from which to choose. It also helps to do more standing than sitting. Standing by itself burns more calories than sitting and improves muscle tone and balance. Try standing for activities that you presently do while sitting, such as talking on the phone or watching TV. One comedian quipped that the answer to the obesity problem in this country would be to require that TVs be powered by treadmills. Inactivity is very detrimental to health and shortens life expectancy. One of my patients frequently tells me that he will aways keep active and then adds, "You know, if I lie down, they will start throwing dirt on top of me."

In addition to maintaining aerobic activity, it is important to do anaerobic muscle-toning exercise. Some may be familiar with osteoporosis, the all-too-common loss of calcium from bones, or its milder form, osteopenia. Fewer are aware of sarcopenia, the age-related loss of muscle mass, yet the statistics for the latter are disturbing.[1] Most of us reach our maximum muscle mass around age thirty and maintain it fairly well until our sixties. Then, unless we take deliberate efforts to reverse the trend, we start losing about 1 percent of our muscle mass each year. Of even greater concern: this loss rises 2 percent per year in our seventies and doubles during each subsequent decade so that it reaches 8 percent per year in our nineties.[2] It does not take much of a math whiz to recognize how much we have left when we get truly old. We must do some muscle-strengthening exercise throughout our lives. This can be done with a set of inexpensive dumbbells or walking with wrist weights. Do not do it the way one of my patients suggested: "I walk each day with my husband—he's a dumbbell! Is that enough?"

35

In addition to doing aerobic and anaerobic exercise, we should stretch and find ways to intentionally improve balance. Group-exercise activities such as Tai Chi or Pilates are excellent for these purposes. While traveling in Asia I have been impressed by seeing many elderly folks outdoors in the early morning doing Tai Chi as a group.

Diet

It is tough to know which is more important for maintaining good health: diet or exercise. There is no question, though, that pre-scribing the best diet is the more difficult to do. Part of the problem is that so many pet theories are touted that have little or no scientific basis.[3] It is further complicated because the problem with diet is more often a lack of will than a lack of knowledge. Most of us know that a healthy diet is heavy on fruits and veggies, rich in fiber but otherwise low in starches (especially sugar and high-fructose corn syrup), moderate in protein, and low in fat. Yet eating this way can be challenging. It can be more expensive and is contrary to the way we were raised. Besides, this type of diet does not include our comfort foods and may be more difficult to prepare tastefully. Yet to be good stewards of the bodies God has given to us, we can and indeed must get our eating act together. I have found that the simplest and best solution is to control the portions that we eat and eliminate snacks and high-calorie beverages. I encourage people to identify their snack weaknesses and to stop buying them. It is easier to resist temptation in the grocery store than in the kitchen. As to portion control, I make several suggestions:

- Eat on a lunch plate, not a dinner plate, and take no second helpings.
- Never finish your dinner at a restaurant. Ask for a take-home box and put the extra food in it before you start eating, not after you are full.
- Stop eating when you are full, not when you have finished all of your food.

- Eat one-course meals; if you have a salad, make it your whole meal and no desserts.
- Drink two big glasses of water before you eat and drink water as your beverage with your meals.
- Avoid all beverages with sweeteners and be aware that artificial sweeteners make you hungrier and do not help you lose weight.
- Eat some denser foods such as nuts before you sit down to eat a large meal.
- Include more fiber in your diet. For years I have used a psyllium powder such as a generic form of Metamucil to get more fiber in my diet. A tablespoon prior to eating is a wonderful way to suppress the appetite.
- Drastically reduce your carbohydrate and sugar intake; they stimulate the secretion of insulin, which makes you hungrier.
- Chew your food well and eat slowly, putting your fork down between each bite.
- Concentrate on eating vegetables; they are often more filling than other foods.

In spite of these suggestions, many people still find it very difficult to achieve portion control. For the motivationally challenged, a group program such as Weight Watchers can be helpful.

Christians often ask my opinion on fasting as a means of weight loss. I do not recommend this, even though I believe strongly in fasting for spiritual reasons. In that context, it is a means of controlling the desires of the flesh in ways that allow us to find our

> STRATEGY
> Find out your ideal weight and lay out a plan to achieve it.

greater satisfaction in God. From a medical point of view, prolonged (more than twenty-four hours) fasting takes a toll on our bodies and should not be used for nonspiritual ends.

Beyond weight control, there are two other aspects of good nutrition that we should consider: salt and cholesterol. We hear a lot about the problems associated with salt and are cautioned not to go overboard on its use. Still, only certain people need to be particularly concerned about their salt intake: many of those with hypertension and those with fluid-retaining conditions such as heart failure and kidney or liver disease. Most of us do not need to severely limit our use of salt. Cholesterol is a more pervasive problem. There are good data showing that the better your cholesterol level, the lower your risk of heart attack or stroke.

There are two numbers in the cholesterol test results (a lipid panel) to focus on. These are the LDL (bad) and HDL (good) cholesterol levels. The government guidelines recommend that the LDL be kept less than 130 for the general population and less than one hundred for those with established hardening of the arteries (having had a heart attack or stroke) and those with several other risk factors such as diabetes. Many cardiologists encourage their patients to try to obtain an LDL of seventy, hoping that the cholesterol already deposited in arteries will actually shrink. Rarely can cholesterol that low be obtained without taking medications. Anyone needing to lower their LDL level should attempt to do so by dieting before using medications. They should limit the intake of animal-based fat (red meats, high milk-fat dairy products), restrict cooking oils (other than olive, peanut, or canola), and avoid baked goods high in saturated fat. It is also helpful to consume more nuts, soy, oats, barley, and ocean-raised fish such as salmon.

To intelligently manage your cholesterol level, you will need to consider how low it needs to be. I have many high-cholesterol patients—even as high as 160—with no other risk factors for heart disease whom I do not encourage to take medications. I do encourage them to follow a low-cholesterol diet. A useful tool to help make the decision about using drugs for cholesterol is an Internet site called Framingham Risk Analysis. When you enter your age, cholesterol readings, and blood pressure, the program will give you your risk of having a heart attack or stroke within the next ten years. High-cholesterol visitors to this site might wish to enter their numbers and then, for purposes of comparison, enter some really good numbers to determine how having better cholesterol levels might lower their risk.

I have seen numerous people on cholesterol-lowering drugs who, before starting treatment, had a less than 5 percent risk. After treatment, the risk has dropped to about 3 percent. What intrigues me is how individuals respond to those differences. They smile and say, "Wow, that is a 40 percent reduction. I want to stay on the drug." Others say, "No way. That risk is so small without medications that I want to stop treatment." Personally, I would side with the second group, but I like the fact that they are making their own decision. A low HDL is also a significant risk factor. Unfortunately, drug therapy is not very effective at raising an HDL. What does help is to increase the amount of aerobic exercise.

It seems that almost every day I see a patient who has heard about some particular diet that promises wonderful results for weight loss or better health. It has been my observation that if there are any benefits to these fad diets, they are experienced by only a minority. If they ask my opinion, I will frequently tell them that I do not see any danger in the diet, but if they do not see the promised results in a reasonable period of time, it is not worth staying with it. There are times when some of these fad diets may actually be dangerous, and it is worth checking them out with your physician.

There is also great interest in a wide range of diet supplements. Some of these are made from regular foods in which many of the nutritional values have been concentrated and purified. Using these can be effective. That said, I am skeptical of most nonfood-based supplements for which specific health claims are made. The amount of research demonstrating their efficacy is usually very scant, there are rarely studies of statistical significance proving their safety, and some may actually be harmful. For people taking prescription drugs, there are almost no studies looking at the interactions between these supplements and prescribed medications. I personally feel that the Lord made our food supply in such a way that a balanced diet gives us what we need, and when we take supplements by themselves, we may miss nutrients necessary for their safe metabolism.[4]

There are two supplements that I frequently recommend. One is a multiple vitamin for anyone who is not able to get a well-balanced diet. The other is calcium combined with vitamin D. Most female adults over fifty should be getting at least fifteen hundred milligrams of calcium a day and men about one thousand milligrams, through eating either dairy products or a supplement. Unless you are in the sun for at least an hour a week, you should take the equivalent of eight hundred units of vitamin D each day. Living in Chicago, I take five thousand units once a week from the first of November to the first of May.

Get Enough Rest

I have found that people rarely think about appropriate rest as being on a par with diet and exercise when it comes to keeping healthy or controlling weight. I am convinced it is and that most people do not get enough. Rest comes in two forms: our daily sleep and appropriate times away from the stresses of life. Sleep is critical. If you wonder if you are getting enough, ask yourself if you are sleepy while doing engaging activities during the day. If you fall asleep during a good sermon on Sunday morning, chances are that you are not getting enough sleep. Sleep deprivation often contributes to overeating and obesity since lack of sleep inhibits the hormonal signals that tell us it is time to stop eating.

Some take adequate time to sleep but find that restful sleep evades them. Frequent trips to the bathroom, sleep apnea, or lack of a quiet room in which to relax can contribute. Shift work can be very detrimental to good sleep. Many of these situations can be helped either by a primary-care physician or by a sleep specialist.

It is much wiser to approach sleep problems by seeking the root cause than by taking sleeping pills.

In the opposite sense, I find that many seniors often have trouble sleeping because they want more sleep than they need. They may take long naps in the day and then are not able to sleep at night. Others may get bored and go to bed too early and then complain that they wake up too soon. They may go to bed at 8:00 p.m. and are frustrated when they waken at 3:00 a.m. I remind them that we cannot force our bodies to get more sleep than we need and that getting too much sleep may make us feel lethargic and unmotivated.

Ben was in the other day, asking for a sleeping pill. As we talked, he told me that he goes to bed at 7:30 p.m. and watches TV until 10:00. He then sleeps fitfully until 6 a.m., finding those nighttime hours long and distressing. He then sleeps soundly from 6:00 until 9:00 a.m., often not getting up until noon. He regularly takes a two-hour afternoon nap. No wonder he can't sleep at night! We concluded that he did not need a sleeping pill but something to keep him busy during the day.

Besides getting enough sleep, we need to get away from the cares of our lives and enjoy some quiet and peace. Believing this is true, I have for many years taken Tuesday as a day off from my office. It gives me time to do other things, often including a long run. As a result, I feel less

> **STRATEGY**
> Consider whether you are getting enough sleep and time away.

pressured the rest of the week. The biblical precedent of a Sabbath, taking one day out of seven to be renewed, is wise. In today's busy world we also do well to take several weeks off each year, if we are able.

When we do not have time to get proper rest, I suspect it is because we are filling our lives with activities that God has not called us to do. The psalmist wrote, "It is in vain that you rise up early and go late to rest, eating the bread of anxious toil; for he gives to his beloved sleep" (Ps. 127:2).

Avoid Unsafe Behaviors

Most of the time, we need to use our common sense to avoid unsafe practices. We don't need to be told not to smoke, to avoid excessive use of alcohol, and to wear our seat belts, bike helmets, or other protective gear when they are necessary. I wish that using a cane or walker did not have such negative associations for many of my patients. Regular use of such aids can help prevent broken hips or other injuries.

Seek Good Medical Care

CHOOSING A PHYSICIAN

I believe good medical care starts with finding a primary-care physician who is well trained, compassionate, easy to relate to, and shares your basic philosophy of medicine. Before you choose a new physician, do your homework. Try to get some referrals from friends. If you are new to a community I suggest that you find a nurse who can

STRATEGY
Determine your unsafe behaviors.

recommend a physician and then check out him or her on the Internet. Be sure to notice his specialty, whether he is board certified, where he did his training, and how long he has been in practice. Also, try to discover his theory of practicing medicine. Primary-care physicians, whether they are family practitioners or internists, will have different philosophies. Some will look on themselves as the quarterback of the team. They will refer you to various specialists who will give most of the care. Others will see themselves as offering a medical home, i.e., a single place where you can get most of your care. They view specialists as consultants who give advice but do not do the primary management. Frankly, I prefer the latter. I tell my patients that, without a doubt, the cardiologist knows more about their heart than I do; but I know more about them as people, a great asset when treating them.

I appreciate patients who schedule a first appointment to "meet and greet." I would suggest some questions you may want to ask potential physicians if you cannot find the answer in other ways:

What is their philosophy for referrals? Do they expect most of your problems to be referred to specialists, or will they provide most of the care?

Do they prefer to manage chronic conditions with medications or with lifestyle changes?

If you are a Christian, explain that your relationship with God is very important to you. Can they respect that? You may even ask if they ever pray with or for patients.

What arrangements does the office have for providing emergency care?

If you require hospitalization, will the physician visit you, or will a full-time hospital physician be in charge?

Many of my patients are Christians, and I find it a joy to serve these fellow believers. They appreciate having a doctor who recognizes God's hand in healing and is willing to pray for them. Personally, however, I would rather have a caring and competent non-Christian physician than choose a doctor simply because he or she is a believer.

PREVENTATIVE CARE

Medicine as a profession is placing greater emphasis these days on prevention. It's about time. Many insurance policies now offer a yearly wellness visit without requiring any payment from the patient. This provides an opportunity to discuss many of the suggestions presented in this chapter with your physician. It also allows you to have your routine vaccinations updated, an important part of maintaining good health. I find it unfortunate that so many people refuse vaccinations, especially flu shots. These shots are very safe, and getting them not only benefits you but also may offer protection to others. Thinking of others in this way is a very "Christian" thing to do.

MEDICATIONS

Medications are available for many conditions, and we must look on them as a gift that God has given to us to defeat many of the illnesses that are part of living in a fallen world. After all, any healing is done by God, whether he uses medicines or not. When I write a prescription, I frequently ask my patients if they ever bow and give thanks for their food. Many say they do. I then ask them if, when they pray, they ever add the phrase "and please bless it to my body's use." Again, many do. I end by suggesting that they give thanks to God for their medicine and ask him to "bless it to their body's use."

Conversely, many drugs are overused. We tend to think we can treat any problem with a pill. Yet many illnesses could be more effectively dealt with through lifestyle changes, which are less expensive and have fewer side effects. I often quote one of my partners, who loves to say, "Medicines are poisons with a few good side effects." Of course, however, there are many situations in which medications are indicated, and we should continue to use them as part of being good stewards of the bodies God has entrusted to us.

Often patients fail to take their medications

STRATEGY
Review your use of medications. Are you using them as a good steward should?

regularly. Even more troubling is how few of them are willing to acknowledge that to their physician. They say they are taking their pills every day, yet they fail to refill their prescriptions. Skipping one's medication is like wearing a seat belt for only part of a trip.

If you fail to take your medicines regularly, I urge you to discuss that with your doctor and give him or her the chance to address the issues involved. If finances are a barrier, there might be a less expensive option. If your problem is remembering to take a medication three times a day, your doctor might prescribe a once-a-day alternative.

Another major problem with medications is that some of them are addicting, particularly sedatives and opium-related painkillers. Prescription drug addiction is a massive problem in the United States. I cannot throw stones, for I have had patients acquire such addictions while under my care. Prescription addictions can occur when the doctor prescribes a stronger dose than is necessary or allows a patient to stay on a medication longer than necessary. One of the consequences of addictive painkillers is that over time they lead to depression and reduced pain tolerance. As a result, patients want stronger and more frequent drugs. By far the best solution for this situation is to never let it get started. If you need a strong painkiller for an acute situation, take as little as possible and get off it as soon as you can. Something nonaddicting such as acetaminophen (Tylenol), ibuprofen (Advil), or naproxen (Aleve) can be very effective. In situations where pain is intractable, it may be best to see a pain specialist.

SURGERY

Surgery can play a significant role in maintaining good health. Common geriatric surgeries include hip and knee replacements. I have had patients with severe joint problems who were literally imprisoned in their homes and forced into inactivity while their muscles deteriorated for lack of exercise. After joint replacement they became active again, not only free of pain but healthier overall and able to serve the Lord in new and productive ways. Just as I try to pray with patients before surgery, I often bow with them afterward to thank God for a good surgical outcome.

The time to consider joint replacement is not necessarily when you are having pain but when the pain begins to interfere with your ability to function. The decision whether to have surgery is an individual one, and many factors must be considered before concluding that the potential benefit outweighs the risks involved. Rarely have I seen anyone regret their choice to pursue surgery.

CANCER

When it comes to cancer, be diligent with screening tests and pursue early and aggressive treatment. Most of us are procrastinators, which can be devastating when dealing with cancer. To care well for our bodies, we will faithfully submit to cancer-screening procedures such as mammograms and colon cancer screening and, in our younger years, prostate exams and pap smears. Most importantly, we will not ignore symptoms that could indicate cancer.

Health: A Blessing from God

Good physical health is a blessing from God. We should never take it for granted but should thank God daily for our health and take care of our bodies as temples of the Holy Spirit, for our bodies are not ours—they belong to God. If we understand that life is not about us but about God's glory, we will want to pursue health and endeavor to use it to do things that will bring God glory. That, after all, is the reason we want to stay healthy—making good use of our bodies. All too often, we think in terms of preserving our health so we can enjoy long years on this earth. That is rather short-sighted, for using our health to advance God's eternal kingdom is much more important than simply prolonging life on earth.

I have chosen to deal with the physical as the first area of wellness because it is a key topic that many are thinking about. The reality of good physical health, however, is that even for those in the best shape, it will be fleeting, and of all the wellness domains we are considering, it is the most likely to elude us. The message of *Wellness for the Glory of God* is that we can continue to be well even as our physical health deteriorates. Wellness is not defined by what our bodies look like or what they can do. When considered from the perspective of each of the other domains of life, wellness can be much more fulfilling and deeply satisfying.

Questions for Reflection and Discussion

What is your current weight?_____ What would you say is your ideal weight?_____

How many hours a week are you engaged in brisk walking or other physical activity?_____

What would your goal be?_____

Do you do any muscle training with weights?_____

Are you stretching?_____

What do you do to improve balance?_____

How would you grade your diet? (A, B, C, D, or F)

Vegetables:_____

Fruits:_____

Low-fat dairy products:_____

How much of your meat intake is: high-fat red meats_____; low-fat red meats_____; chicken or turkey_____; fish_____; vegetable protein (tofu, etc.)_____

How many hours of sleep do you average each night? _____

Is that too little, too much, or just right? Circle the correct answer.

Circle the screening tests that you are due for: mammogram, pap smear, colon cancer screening, cholesterol.

Prayer

Lord,

You have given me a body and want me to take the best care of it that I can. I recognize that you are in control over everything, including my physical health. I know you have commanded me to be a good steward of my body. Being weak, I so often give in to temptations to do things that do not promote my physical well-being. I pray that you will give me the wisdom to know how to care for my body as well as the will power to do it. Allow me to use the strength you give me to do things for you and to set a good example for others. Most of all, I want you to be glorified through my physical health. I pray this for my own good and for your glory.

Amen

3

Mental Wellness

DEVELOP YOUR MIND

Jessie has always been mentally sharp and still is at eighty-six. She is a diabetic and has a bad heart and poor circulation, so she needs a walker to get around and can no longer drive. Even though I'd known she is a reader who keeps up with current events, you can imagine my surprise when she told me that she has been riding the county bus each week to the community college for an introductory computer course. That's what I call "developing your mind." Now, I admit, Jessie is an exception. Not all of us will be able to follow her example, because our intellectual prowess usually deteriorates with age. But since some of that decline might be avoidable, we should be proactive to preserve as much of our intellectual function as possible. Refraining from exercising our minds can lead to a mental lethargy similar to the lethargy our bodies feel when we do not exercise them. Choosing to do the rigorous thinking we are capable of will maximize our intellectual function as we age. Yet this does not come naturally to most seniors; too many let their minds languish.

Keep Sharp

In some instances dementia will occur and, try as we might, there is only so much we can do to deter it. Many of my older patients live in fear of dementia. Since I have a strong family history of dementia, there is part of me that fears it too. I, like many others, hate the thought of losing my mental capacity, giving up control, and becoming dependent on others. For too long we may have associated our value with our IQs and ability to be independent. But that is not how God sees us. In order to be anywhere near well in the context of dementia we must accept the loss of our intellectual function graciously, submitting to what God has ordained for us. I have honestly seen some people with dementia who could be considered well. Whether that resulted from choices they made or was simply God's grace, I am not sure. At the same time, I have seen many with dementia who would not be considered anywhere near well.

This is the second thing we must do if we wish to stay well to the glory of God—improve our minds. We start with what may be the easiest: the strategies we can use to develop our minds while they still work reasonably well. The greater challenge will come as we consider strategies to promote wellness even when our minds fail.

The Healthy Brain

God has blessed all who are able to read this book with a reasonably healthy brain. Just as we are to be stewards of the bodies he has given us, so we are to be stewards of our minds. Maintaining our mental abilities does not come naturally, nor will one approach help everyone. It may be challenging and will require deliberate planning and discipline, for the old adage, "If you don't use it, you lose it," is particularly true of our minds. Following are some suggestions to follow.

Read as much as you can. Jeff at ninety-six is still an avid reader. A retired pastor, he maintains an interest in current events, and each week he devours both *Time* and *Newsweek*. He is fascinating to talk with. When he goes down for dinner in his independent-living community, there is always someone who invites him to share the meal together. But his reading does not stop with current events. Reading widely, Jeff constantly stretches his brain and impresses others with how much he retains from what he reads.

Christians do well to spend some time each day reading the Scriptures. Consider a reading program in which you will read the Bible through in a year, or take your time and do it in two years. One program I have used is that from Robert Murray M'Cheyne, which is available from many different sources.[1] For me, it is not enough to read; I need to stop and think about what I have read. Paul's instruction to Timothy was to "think over what I say, for the Lord will give you understanding in everything" (2 Tim. 2:7). Then, if I am going to truly understand what the Lord is saying to me, I need to jot down my thoughts in a journal or diary.

In addition, when I read other books, I record my reflections on the blank pages at the end of the book. That forces me to understand what the author is saying and think through how it applies to me. If I don't pause to think and write, much of my time reading is wasted.[2]

Memorizing Scripture can help us keep our mental faculties. I have a number of older friends who regularly do this. They recognize that it is not as easy as it used to be. One of my friends complained that memorizing Scripture was like pouring water through a sieve. Then she smiled and quipped, "But have you ever seen a dirty sieve?"

Keep learning new things. How many times in your earlier years have you said, "That's fascinating, and sometime I want to take the time to learn something about that"? Well, now may be the time. Is it a field of science or music? Have you thought of learning to play an instrument or a new card game? You can listen to college lectures on CD or watch them on DVD. What about carefully studying a book of the Bible that you have never gotten into? When you meet Ezekiel in heaven, will you two be able to have an intelligent conversation? Or will he be a total stranger? The possibilities for mental exercise are endless.

In addition to these activities you can pursue on your own, develop your mind by getting involved in a social group with people who like to think. Consider joining a book club or going to a play with someone and discussing it afterward. A group of six of my retired patients meet at a local restaurant twice a week for coffee and, according to them, "solve the problems of the world." I also know of a group of about twenty seniors who meet at a restaurant once a week for a Bible study. These folks are sharpening their brains for the present and doing a lot to preserve their intellects for the future. They are also double tasking, for as they are sharpening their own minds, they are serving others by encouraging them to think and express themselves.

Two other common ways for seniors to sharpen their brains while serving others are to maintain an active prayer ministry and constantly encourage others. Keep lists of prayer requests, update them, and pray through those lists regularly. Buy boxes of note cards and send regular notes of encouragement to your friends, whether they are younger or older. The recipients will appreciate them, and it will be of great help to you—a true win-win.

Do not confine your social circle to just Christians or to those who think the same way you do. Spend time with people who view the world differently and allow them to challenge your thinking. Some of these social connections can be done from home. Join the modern world by turning on your computer, and open a Facebook page on which you can record your thoughts and correspond with your friends.

Use TV and other entertainment wisely. Much of what is available on TV is amusing but requires little thinking (the word *a-muse* literally means *no thinking.*)

Thankfully, that is not true of all that is on TV. If you are going to spend time watching something, consider inviting

> **STRATEGY**
> Determine to stretch your brain by continuing to think and learn.

someone to join you and then talk about what you have seen. It is amazing how valuable this can be.

Much of the ability to think and reflect depends on our preserving our sensory input to the greatest extent possible. For some, that will require getting hearing aids, having cataracts removed, or getting treatment for glaucoma or macular degeneration. If your eyesight does not allow you to read, take advantage of some of the electronic media available to keep feeding your mind. There are all kinds of audio books at the local library.

Unfortunately, developing our brains is not the default of our culture, as it takes both effort and energy. There is a lot of gray-headed brainpower going to waste. Don't let it be yours.

The Failing Brain: Three Categories

Though I love to be upbeat and emphasize the positive when talking about mental wellness, I must spend the majority of this chapter dealing with the challenges that might be encountered when the brain begins to fail. First, I must acknowledge that the failing brain can present a definite paradox. It can lead to some of the greatest challenges we will face in this life and cause some of our greatest heartaches. At the same time it may represent a wonderful opportunity for God to do his transforming work in our character and prove that his grace is sufficient for any trial.

Let me define some of the concepts related to memory loss. There are three categories, which lie on a spectrum:

Benign	Mild	
Senescent—————————	Cognitive—————————	Dementia
Forgetfulness	Impairment	

These three categories are not entirely distinct, and sometimes it is difficult to know where one transitions into the other.

Benign senescent forgetfulness is typified by recent memory loss and is a part of normal aging. It is seen in healthy brains and will happen to all of us if we live long enough. I jokingly tell my patients that there are two groups of seniors: those who acknowledge their memory loss and those who deny it. We may be able to talk about where we celebrated our anniversary thirty years ago but may not be quite sure what we ate for dinner last night or the name of our neighbor. In this category of memory loss, problems are confined to the memory and associated word recall; the other areas of neurological function and our basic personality structure are still intact. If we are able to recognize our forgetfulness and make allowances for it, it is clear that we are still on the left side of the dementia spectrum and dealing only with benign senescent forgetfulness.

Mild cognitive impairment (MCI) is the most difficult of the three categories to recognize. Within the spectrum of cognitive decline, this condition lies in the gray zone between a forgetful healthy brain and dementia. Here the memory loss is more severe, and problems show up in at least one other area of brain function. The individual may demonstrate poor judgment or a change in personality. There may be loss of coordination, physical strength, or organizational skills. In spite of these changes, a person will still function adequately in the community and be quite independent. As a result, these problems may be noticed only by those who are closest to him. The individual may be able to successfully bluff and live in denial.

Dementia will be the end result for some of those with MCI (about 12 percent in any one year will move from MCI to dementia). At that point, they will show deficits in several areas of neurological function, and the difficulties they had in MCI will typically become worse. Poor judgment may lead to tragic mistakes or weakness, and lack of coordination may lead to falls. Those with moderate to severe dementia will no longer be able to live independently. Though it is not an accurate method, one simple way to recognize those with dementia is that they tend to forget that they forget. I am not as worried about the seniors who come to the office and tell me that they are concerned that they are getting demented. They tell me a story about how they put their keys in the wrong pocket and forgot where they put them, or how they went shopping and got home without the milk they went for. I admit to them that I do those things too. I tell them that either they are probably okay or they need a new doctor. Conversely, I did worry about the patient who was found by police fifty miles from home. When his daughter explained that he'd gotten lost, he grunted and said, "Don't listen to her. That never happened!" He wasn't lying—he had simply forgotten that it had happened.

> **STRATEGY**
>
> If you feel that you are losing some of your normal brain function, review the suggestions to preserve a healthy brain, to maintain the abilities you have left.

Mild Cognitive Impairment (MCI)

A small but significant group of people with MCI may have some correctable disease that treatment can delay or stop the progression to dementia. For this reason, I usually recommend a complete physical exam when it is clear that the memory problems are getting worse. This includes tests for thyroid, Vitamin B12, and some type of brain imaging, ideally an MRI; if an MRI is not possible, a CAT scan can be used to look for a problem within the brain itself. Many times these studies show atrophy, which is generalized shrinking of the brain. I need to reassure the patient and family that this is a sign of aging, not necessarily dementia.

Once MCI occurs, there are no medications or proven strategies to assure it will not progress to dementia. Rather than seeking a way to stop it, we must look for what may slow its progression. Here we go back to the basics. Studies have shown that aerobic exercise, such as walking thirty minutes a day,[3] and eating a healthy diet low in fats and sugars while high in plant-sourced foods, such as vegetables and soy-based products, can help.[4] There is reasonably good evidence that eating certain antioxidant-rich foods such as blueberries (and many other fruits) and red beans slows the deterioration.[5] As we've noted already, it helps to keep using all the intellectual capacity we still have and to stay involved with other people.[6]

As soon as MCI is recognized, it is time to consider drug therapy. Admittedly, the drugs available are not as effective as we would like. In fact, the US Food and Drug Administration will allow the manufacturers of the available drugs to claim only that they may slow down the progression of the disease.

> **STRATEGY**
>
> If you are developing symptoms that seem more than benign senescent forgetfulness, do not deny them but pursue medical and legal help.

They cannot claim they will actually reverse the impairment. Nevertheless, the drugs seem to be more effective early in the course of cognitive impairment rather than later. Depression and MCI frequently go together and often contribute to each other. Depression may be more treatable than dementia.

Since MCI has a high probability of developing into dementia, it is wise for those who are moving in this direction to make legal arrangements while they are still competent to do so. These should include reviewing or making both a medical and a financial power of attorney as well as a will and trust agreement.

Dementia

Dementia is common in the elderly population and will become even more common as life expectancy increases. It has been estimated that at age sixty-five, 5 percent of the US population has some form of dementia, and as this group ages, the number will double roughly every seven years so that by age ninety, half will experience dementia. Since not all forms of dementia are the same, it helps to be able to distinguish them. Many of my patients believe all dementia is Alzheimer's disease. It is true that Alzheimer's is the most common type, but it is only one form of dementia. I often explain that dementia is like the word *car*, and Alzheimer's is like a Ford. Alzheimer's makes up about 70 percent of the cases of dementia, but there are other common causes, including multiple strokes and a form of dementia often associated with Parkinson's disease called "Lewy body." In addition, there are a host of other less-common conditions that can lead to dementia. It is helpful to have as careful a diagnosis as possible, because the treatment and prognosis of various causes can vary.

I have learned some about dementia in my medical studies and even more through the experience of my patients, but perhaps I have learned the most through my mother's experience. I had the privilege of being raised in a wonderful Christian home with godly parents. My mother was loving, kind, and well-tempered—always giving to others. At the time of this writing, she is severely de-mented at age ninety-two. She lives in the nursing-home wing of the retirement community where she has been for almost twenty years. Widowed twelve years ago, Mother lived independently for nine years after Dad died, in spite of progressive memory loss, but then she had a series of falls. My siblings and I helped her move to an assisted-living apartment in the retirement community, an arrangement that she graciously accepted. There she continued to be happy and do well until she became irritable and showed some personality change that required a move to the nursing-home wing. Some of her behavior had become totally contrary to that of the mother I have known for sixty-five years. She would strike out at the aides and scream if she had the least discomfort. It was hard to see her like that. Mom usually knew my siblings and me, but sometimes it appeared that she only viewed us as nice strangers to have around.

Though my mother's story is all too common, dementia does not always affect people in the same way. There are times when the sorrow of dementia is experienced more by the loved ones than by the patient. The person who suffers from dementia may be blissfully unaware of the problem, and in such cases, we look on them with pity even though they are quite content.

Biblical Perspectives on Dementia

It has been my habit for many years to seek biblical perspectives on the challenges I have in life. Dementia is not specifically mentioned in the Bible; nevertheless, we find some ideas in Scripture that may help to inform our approach to it. These include the following.

All Human Beings Are Made in God's Image

"So God created man in his own image, in the image of God he created him; male and female he created them" (Gen. 1:27). There is a dignity intrinsic to all humans that sets them apart from the rest of creation. That dignity is not based on our intellect or our ability to accomplish certain tasks. When we lose our mental abilities, we do not lose our status as being made in the image of God. There is something profoundly Godlike even in the most demented person.

We Are to Honor Our Parents

"Honor your father and your mother, that your days may be long in the land that the LORD your God is giving you" (Ex. 20:12). In ancient rabbinic tradition, "to honor" primarily meant taking financial responsibility for parents' welfare. One commentator writes:

> The whole aim of this commandment is to secure positive support for the aging parents from their children, who are themselves assumed to be mature adults. When families lived together in large groups, aging parents who could no longer work were entirely dependent upon their children to support them economically. It is this care of the old that is demanded here.[7]

Jesus's teaching certainly concurs with this. He reprimanded the Pharisees for condoning *Corban*, a legal loophole used to temporarily transfer assets to the temple so that the adult children did not have to use these funds to support their parents (Mark 7:9–13). Paul emphasized this same theme when he wrote, "If anyone does not provide for his relatives, and especially for members of his household, he has denied the faith and is worse than an unbeliever" (1 Tim. 5:8). Of course, honoring our parents should go well beyond financial support and include dealing with them respectfully, lovingly, and kindly. Our Lord commanded: "So whatever you wish that others would do to you, do also to them" (Matt. 7:12).

The Bible Does Not Require Adult Children to Obey Demented Parents

"Children, obey your parents in everything, for this pleases the Lord" (Col. 3:20). It's important to understand the intent of the apostle Paul's command to obey one's parents. I have seen it cause considerable consternation for well-meaning adult children who believe it means they must give in to unrealistic demands of their demented parents. We know that the context of Paul's admonition here deals with young children, since the Greek word Paul uses for "children" refers to little children, not offspring in general. This verse should not be taken to mean that we are obligated to obey all the requests of demented parents. We honor them by carefully considering what they want, but we are not required to strictly obey everything they ask of us.

We Should Selflessly Provide for Those Who Cannot Do for Themselves

"And the King will answer them, 'Truly, I say to you, as you did it to one of the least of these my brothers, you did it to me'" (Matt. 25:40). Surely people who suffer from dementia fall into the category of "the least of these," whom we are instructed to care for. Jesus taught us to "do good . . . expecting nothing in return" (Luke 6:35). Though the context specifically refers to the treatment of enemies, our own families should be treated no less lovingly. True spiritual ministry should not be done with an eye to what we will get in return. This is particularly applicable to the service we provide to those who are demented. We can tirelessly give to them, while they will give little to us in return.

As we give of ourselves to those with significant dementia, we must remember that their world is increasingly contracting, both in time and space. They live primarily in the present tense. They will often not remember the past or be concerned about the future, but they can still enjoy what is done for them in the present. Also, they become less concerned with the world outside and eventually many care only about themselves. Still, we can do many things for them that they can enjoy in the moment, as we will consider later in this chapter.

God Controls All Things to Accomplish His Purpose
"I cry out to God Most High, to God who fulfills his purpose for me" (Ps. 57:2). We can learn two basic lessons in this passage. First, God is in control of this world, and nothing happens apart from his sovereign will. He has a purpose in all that he does. "The LORD will fulfill his purpose for me; your steadfast love, O LORD, endures forever. Do not forsake the work of your hands" (Ps. 138:8). His purpose is always consistent with his steadfast love. At times we may feel forsaken, for it is often hard to discern why he allows dementia. Though we may not have answers and be left wondering, we can still trust that he has a purpose. Moses reminds us, "The secret things belong to the LORD our God, but the things that are revealed belong to us" (Deut. 29:29). Dementia may be one of those secrets that he has chosen not to allow us to understand. We must rest in what he has revealed; he is loving and strong. The second lesson we learn in Psalm 57:2 is that when we are left wondering, we have biblical precedent to cry out to God in our despair,

asking for his strength and comfort as we struggle to trust him to do what is right.

With these biblical perspectives in mind, we now come back to our question, How can someone with dementia be well? To answer this, we must keep in mind the big picture, including the impact of dementia on the life of the individual, the caregivers, the larger community, and the church. In presenting my answer, I admit I can appear overly optimistic, for I am presenting a best-case scenario, which is not the reality for many. Dementia is part of our living in a fallen world; it was not a part of God's original creation. Dementia can be nasty and ugly. Yet God takes the consequences of the fall and uses them to accomplish his overriding purpose—that he himself be glorified. We see that best illustrated in the cross of Jesus and can continue to see that in the challenges we face in our lives today.

The Patient

I have observed several positive things in the lives of patients who are experiencing dementia. First, in the early stages some who have been fiercely independent throughout their lives begin to mellow out. This can be particularly true in a spiritual sense. Individuals who have had no time for the gospel, thinking they could manage without God's help, can become more receptive to their need for a Savior and be willing to trust their eternal well-being to Jesus. Les is a good example. He faithfully went to church with his godly wife all of his adult life but told me it was just to keep her company; he did not really need God's help and had great difficulty believing in a loving God in view of all the suffering in the world. At sixty he began to show more memory problems, and by sixty-five he was really struggling. He commented to me how much he has come to appreciate his wife's being there for him and added how much his faith has come to mean since he now knows he is totally dependent on God for eternal life. As the incapacity from dementia progresses, people like Les may be more open to God and others helping them and develop a meekness and humility that would never have been possible otherwise.

We stereotype dementia and project our own values on the demented, thinking they must be quite miserable. However, I have seen many demented patients who appear quite happy. I have often observed that when I walk into a nursing home and hear laughter, it is invariably coming from the wing where the patients with dementia live. I remember Eva, a retired missionary, who suffered from severe dementia. I would never see her except surrounded by a group of several similarly afflicted patients. She would be slapping her hip and telling a funny story. She was literally the life of the party. No matter that she was telling the same story over and over. Her audience did not care, since they did not remember it anyway. One advantage of dementia is that we never hear an old joke. Dementia can also free the patient from some of the guilt feelings and anxieties that were acquired in earlier years.

The Caregivers

Being the caregiver of a demented person can be fraught with challenges. It is the most common cause of depression in people in their fifties and represents some of the greatest points of need in our culture, especially in our churches. Yet even at the point of desperation, the caregiver can take consolation in the fact that God is in control. He is accomplishing his purpose not only in the life of the patient but also in the life of the caregiver. I often refer to the image that the prophet Isaiah gives us of the potter and the clay: "But now, O LORD, you are our Father; we are the clay, and you are our potter; we are all the work of your hand" (Isa. 64:8). Caregivers often feel like they are being spun around on a potter's wheel; their experience can be a miserable one. But, through it, they are having their rough edges knocked off by a loving God, who is making them into vessels that will bring him glory. I remember Frank, who came to the office after Mary Ellen, his wife of sixty-eight years, died. She experienced progressive dementia for the last five years of her life, and it was very hard on Frank. Yet as he sat in my office sobbing, he said that he did not regret those days because through them the Lord taught him a patience he had never thought he'd have.

As with so many of the difficult times of life we are forced to endure, caregivers don't always look at their plight as Frank did. It is rarely appropriate to try to teach these lessons to people while they are in the midst of their struggle. They don't need a lecture on the theology of suffering; they need our presence, practical help, hugs, prayers, and encouragement. One of the least helpful things we can do when we see a friend overwhelmed with the daily demands of trying to care for someone with dementia is say, "If there is anything I can do, let me know." That may make us feel good, but it puts an additional burden on our friend. In reality it is saying, "Think through all the things you need to do, size up my time, abilities, and interests to see if there is something you feel I would like to do, then try to get hold of me and explain the entire situation." Wouldn't it be better to say, "I see you need to do the wash every other day. How about if I pick up the laundry every Saturday morning and return it cleaned that evening?"

When I see a couple in which one has dementia and the other is the caregiver, I often commend them for fulfilling the promise they made many years before, when they stood before their friends and said, "I take you . . . for richer, for poorer, in sickness and in health, till death do us part." I acknowledge with them that although dementia was not in their minds back then, today they are still doing what they vowed they would. For some, caregiving is not simply a duty to be performed but an opportunity to love. Robertson McQuilkin resigned the presidency of Columbia International University to care for his wife, Muriel, who was afflicted with Alzheimer's. In his letter of resignation he reflected on his role as caregiver:

> Duty . . . can be grim and stoic. But there is more: I love Muriel. She is a delight to me—her childlike dependence and confidence in me, her warm love, occasional flashes of that wit I used to relish so, her happy spirit and tough resilience in the face of her continual distressing frustration. I don't have to care for her. I get to! It is a high honor to care for so wonderful a person [8]

The Community

The larger community, including the church, can benefit from the challenge of dementia. Christians can show how they value all persons by how they respectfully serve their demented fellow human beings. In doing so, they are affirming that people have value because they are made in God's image, not because of what they do. This is a critically important lesson for all believers to learn.

There are many opportunities for the church to be involved in the care of demented patients. All too often, the individuals and their caregivers are marginalized and forgotten. The caregivers desperately need respite that members of the church can provide. Among other things, church members can stay with the patient while the caregiver gets to go out. This practical

STRATEGY

Recognize that amidst all of the frustrations of dementia, God is accomplishing good things.

demonstration of love can be an effective demonstration of God's love and speaks loudly to observers from the non-Christian world. Most chronic-care facilities encourage church groups to provide singing and companionship for patients with dementia. Short-term missions trips can be great, but at times I find it ironic that we will go across the globe to serve in a different culture but will not travel down the street to minister in a local nursing home.

Helping a Demented Person

As dementia progresses, the sufferers may become frustrated by recognizing that they have a problem but not grasping how to deal with it. Also, the caregiver becomes frustrated dealing with someone who seems so different from the person they have known and loved over the years, who now can be unreasonable and childlike. If we are going to come anywhere close to including wellness and dementia in the same sentence, we must be aware of some common challenges we will likely face.

Challenges to Face

DENIAL

Those with early dementia or, even more commonly, patients with minimal cognitive impairment will often deny they have a problem, making it difficult for them to accept treatment or help. John, for example, has clearly been in denial for the past two years. His brother-in-law patiently works with him and attempts to hold things together, but John refuses to admit his needs despite his inability to manage his life. He is oblivious to the deterioration that is obvious to everyone who knows him. He has gotten lost numerous times, is unable to handle his financial affairs, lives by himself in a filthy home, and has very poor nutrition. His family has tried everything, even attempting to practice "tough love" by withdrawing all support from him. Since nothing has worked, they have chosen to be kind, loving, and supportive while expecting that at some point a catastrophe will happen that will force John to accept the help and guidance he needs.

INDEPENDENCE

Since we all want to be independent, our struggle for self-sufficiency often fuels denial. Those becoming demented want to stay in their own home, continue to drive, and manage their own affairs. The very independence that they think is sparing loved ones a lot of work and responsibility is actually making it harder for them. One phrase I frequently use at the office is "the ministry of dependence"—how we help others by not being so fiercely independent. It sometimes helps if we explain the difficulty of helping someone who claims not to need it. In other cases, such explanation seems to fall on deaf ears.

Driving is one form of independence that is difficult to give up. In all honesty, most people with early dementia can drive safely. The problem is typically not accidents but getting lost. I make several suggestions to my patients. First, if they want to keep driving safely, they should frequently drive with another person in the car who can monitor their performance while they keep up their driving skills. They can also get the same results from driver's evaluation programs, which are often sponsored by rehab hospitals and driving schools. Recommendations against driving are often accepted more easily if they come from a professional than from a family member. The more we try to deal with driving and other independence issues in peaceful ways, the more God will be glorified.

ANGER

It is frustrating for people to realize they have dementia, and they might react to it with anger. Such anger is sometimes directed toward the world in general or toward God, but most commonly it is vented toward those they must depend on. Caregivers might have to deal with their own anger, for it is easy to respond to anger by becoming angry in return. That is not always bad. I have seen occasions in which the demented person never caught on to what was being said till the caregiver finally became angry.

I am never one to show much anger, but I recall one experience in which I did. My mother-in-law was living in St. Louis in a retirement community and struggling with the early stages of dementia. She had made many wise choices to accommodate her declining abilities, but my wife, Dorothy, was still making monthly trips from Chicago to St. Louis to check on and help her. Even that was not enough. We had Mother come to our home to visit some of the assisted-living facilities nearby. When we sat down around the kitchen table to discuss the next move, she became entrenched. She enjoyed where she was, she did not need our help, and she was not going to make a move. I became good and angry and laid out for her very clearly all the changes we foresaw happening in her life and why continuing on as she was simply would not work. I doubt if she had ever seen me so upset, but she got the point and agreed to the move. In that situation, good and angry really did go together. Conversely, it is easy for anger to get out of hand, and there is a danger of getting so angry with a demented person that physical abuse results.

DEPRESSION

Many with dementia also suffer from depression. Given their memory problems, counseling is rarely helpful; antidepressant medications may be. Other strategies can help too. For example, depression is reduced when others recognize and show respect for the capacities that depressed people still have. One way to do this is to allow demented patients to make independent decisions, albeit with limited options. For instance, when at an ice cream store, instead of asking, "What flavor do you want?" ask: "Do you want chocolate or vanilla?" Also, give them jobs that they are able to do. Sue was eighty-six with moderate dementia, and we were concerned she was slipping into depression. Then one fall day she came into the office bragging about how many piles of leaves she had raked. She could not remember anything else to tell me, but she was anxious that I know that she could work hard. I am sure that her daughter could have done the job in half the time, but by involving her mother, Sue's daughter allowed Sue the self-respect she deserved, helping to ameliorate her depression.

PERSONALITY CHANGE

One of the most difficult aspects of dementia is the personality change that so often accompanies it. Some of the sweetest, most loving people in the world can become physically, verbally, and emotionally abusive. Whatever has inhibited such responses in years gone by no longer works, and an entirely new personality emerges. There may be little resemblance to the person one has loved and respected for many years. As it did at times with my mother, self-control goes out the window, and patients say and do exactly what first comes to mind. They may have no ability to reason and no insight into the impact that their behavior has on others. When this occurs, they may respond to loving and patient confrontation, but unfortunately this may not have any lasting impact. Interestingly, the opposite will sometimes occur too—some who have always been hard to get along with seem to mellow out and become quite congenial.

INFLEXIBILITY

Change is hard at any age but especially for those with dementia. Significant changes should be minimized. I have seen large families try to move their demented parent from one home to another each month—a recipe for disaster. Even moving to and from the hospital often leads to a major setback. When any of my demented patients are in a nursing home, I do my utmost to keep them there rather than sending them to the hospital, where the disruption in daily routine so often leads to more confusion and agitation.

LONELINESS

One of the most beneficial things we can provide patients who have dementia is our presence. In the earlier stages of the disease, we can plan to do meaningful activities with them. It is important to identify the interests they have had in the past and allow them to experience those pleasures again. If they were readers, try reading to them. Artists may enjoy seeing art or even doing some simple art projects with you. My mother-in-law was an avid gardener and loved flowers. Before the dementia became too disabling, she loved to go to a nearby garden and enjoy the beauty. During the later stages of dementia, all that may be necessary is your being with the patient. In very late dementia, the individual may be like a three-month-old. A baby cannot articulate anything but certainly derives comfort from knowing that Mom is there. Sometimes there is nothing more meaningful to them than to be touched and reminded God still loves them.

LIMITED COMMUNICATION

One key to engaging those with a demented brain is to reach into their past to help them recall pleasant memories. When possible, spend generous time talking about the earlier years of their lives. Ask about their childhood, their wedding, or the birth of their children. Talk through old picture albums or provide other links to the past. Read them stories about things that occurred in their youth. Give them things to hold that they can associate with their past, allowing them to relive past pleasures. I have seen a number of older women derive great comfort from holding a baby doll or stuffed animal. Pets can provide a connection with the past and be calming, and music can be particularly soothing.

Just as it is difficult for us to penetrate through the wall of dementia in ways that are meaningful to the patients, it is equally difficult for them to communicate with us. One has to be very perceptive to understand their intent. When they spit out food, they are not simply trying to be difficult. Often they are saying, "I don't care for this. Please give me something else." Withdrawal or increased agitation may indicate discomfort from constipation or a bladder infection. When disruptive behaviors are seen, it is essential that we try to discern what is precipitating them before we respond.

Though it may be difficult to communicate with the mind of a demented person, it may still be possible to engage the spirit. The Bible teaches that in some way our spirit is distinct from our minds. Paul made this point when he wrote: "I will pray with my spirit, but I will pray with my mind also; I will sing praise with my spirit, but I will sing with my mind also" (1 Cor. 14:15). Our comforter, the Holy Spirit, may continue to work in a demented brain. Believers, even those with severe dementia, may be engaged when we pray with and for them. Some will be able to quote Scripture. Try starting a verse (in a Bible translation familiar to the patient) and let them finish it. Christian music also has a transforming role on our spirits. I have frequently seen agitated patients quieted by hymns they had sung years ago. Prior to her dementia my mother would often be asked to sit with the dying in her retirement community. I recall mom telling me, "I never know what to say, so I just quietly hold their hands and sing to them." I don't think she could have done better. If you cannot sing, you can quote the lyrics of the old hymns of the faith. I have occasionally shared Communion with demented people and have found that this helps them remember the Lord's death on their behalf.

CAREGIVER FATIGUE

Perhaps the greatest burden of dementia is the personal sacrifice of the caregiver. I have already mentioned that, all too often, demented patients are hardest on the one they are most dependent on. They can even get to the point of being downright mean. More than once I have seen a loving daughter driven to tears by the demented mother who lives with her. Then when her brother visits, the mom is absolutely delightful, and he cannot understand his sister's complaints. Another trait of the demented that can be extremely annoying for the caregiver is the day-to-day variation in their ability. One day a father can carry on a good conversation whereas the next day he is totally confused. Because it takes a lot of mental energy to pull the brain together, the patient can no longer do it on a consistent basis. At times the patient will be more motivated to do so; other times he will not. This makes the caregiver's day-to-day planning exasperating.

Caregiver fatigue is a huge issue that never receives enough emphasis. It may lead to totally unacceptable results, including depression in the caregiver, unsanitary conditions, and abuse of the demented person. An excellent book titled *The 36-Hour Day* is a most helpful resource for understanding what caregiving involves.[9] The title sums it up well: caregivers need to reach out for help when they need it; they should not try to be heroes.

Where to Provide Care

The residence of those with dementia is an important aspect of their well-being. The best and most obvious option is remaining in their own home with live-in help. That offers huge advantages. But finding the right helpers may be difficult, and paying them can be expensive. Living with one of their children is a possible option, but this places a huge burden on the host family and can be lonely and unsafe for the patient if help is not present 24/7. It requires great sacrifice

STRATEGY

If you are caring for someone with dementia, recognize the challenges and do not be embarrassed to ask your church for help.

on the part of caregivers and their families, although there are rewards as well. Such an arrangement works well only if the patient is aware enough to appreciate the sacrifices being made on his or her behalf. When demented persons no longer recognize where they are, it may well be time to relocate them to a carefully chosen chronic-care facility.

Emily is a case in point. Her daughter, Marge, cared for Emily at home through the early stages of dementia while still going to work each day. After a year or so, Emily was increasingly agitated later in the day, did not sleep at night, and constantly yelled out for help. She was totally disoriented and did not recognize her daughter. Finally, with much misgiving Marge moved her to a nursing home, where she lived for the last six months of her life, and as far as we could tell, she seemed more contented there. Too often I have heard elderly patients asking their children to promise never to place them in a nursing home, but I counsel these children never to agree to such a promise.

Treatment of Dementia

Unfortunately, pharmacologic treatment for dementia is in its infancy. Still, if medications are not started early in the course of dementia, at the stage of MCI, they should be considered once dementia is full-blown. I have seen medications be of significant help in a few patients, and I generally recommend they be given a try. Even if they do not improve the memory, they will at times help curb some of the negative behavior associated with dementia. On the other hand, if the dementia drugs do not seem to help, and especially if they cause side effects, I feel no obligation to continue them.

Two other things that have proven effective are formal memory training (often available only in a large dementia clinic) and the supplement melatonin. Many other commonly used supplements, such as folic acid, vitamin B12 (when there is no deficiency identified), ginkgo biloba, and vitamin E, have been shown to have no benefit.[10]

When treating dementia, it becomes necessary to consider how aggressive we should be when other medical conditions arise. There are no easy answers. In formulating an approach, we should first keep in mind that dementia, just like heart failure or cancer, is a progressive, terminal disease. Death may not be immediate, but eventually the patient will succumb to either the dementia or complications related to it. Given that fact, it is appropriate to treat conditions when easily done and to promote comfort for the patient.

On the other hand, as dementia progresses and quality of life deteriorates, there is no obligation to treat every problem that develops, especially when the treatment itself will cause considerable pain or suffering. For example, in the case of my mother, with her severe dementia, family members have agreed that she

> **STRATEGY**
> In the event that you become demented, make sure your family knows how much life-sustaining care you will want once you are unable to decide for yourself.

will not be hospitalized or given antibiotics if she develops severe pneumonia that will rapidly prove fatal. If she gets a bladder infection that will not kill her but merely cause discomfort, we want her to receive antibiotics. Also, we will avoid chemotherapy or surgery for a condition in which she can be kept comfortable in other ways.

In the later stages of dementia, as death approaches, the patient frequently stops eating and dies of complications from malnutrition. In such cases, I do not believe it is appropriate to employ a feeding tube. It is not uncomfortable to die without artificial nutrition and hydration unless the mouth becomes dry; additionally, forced feeding often leads to unwanted complications such as diarrhea and bedsores. Using feeding tubes in this context may only prolong the dying process.[11] As the end of a demented person's life draws near, it is frequently more appropriate to pursue hospice care rather than aggressive, life-prolonging treatment.

Mental Wellness

To be mentally well, we should try to preserve our intellectual abilities as much as we can and determine to trust God's providence while doing our best when we begin to lose those abilities. Can wellness and dementia coexist? The answer is the proverbial "yes, but ..." Yes, it is possible; but it requires a great deal of effort, self-sacrificing love, careful planning, the right living situation, proper use of medical care, a profound trust in God, and the caregiver's receiving needed help and support.

Questions for Reflection and Discussion

What are you doing to develop your mental capacities?

_____

_____

_____

_____

What *could* you be doing to develop your mental capacities?

_____

_____

_____

_____

If you feel you are showing signs of mental deterioration that go beyond normal forgetfulness, what steps should you be taking?

_____

_____

_____

_____

On what basis would you say there is value to a person with dementia?

_____

_____

_____

_____

If you suffered from dementia, would you want the following treatments ?

	Yes	No
Open-heart surgery	_____	_____
Antibiotics for pneumonia	_____	_____
Pain killers	_____	_____
Feeding tube	_____	_____
Have you discussed these with your family?	_____	_____

Prayer

Heavenly Father,

About the last thing I want before you take me home is to suffer from dementia. Help me to do everything possible to preserve the ability of my mind to think and to serve you. But if dementia is in my future, help me to know that you are loving and strong. You will not allow me to face any difficulty without equipping me to handle it in a way that will bring honor and glory to you. Help me to trust you in this, as in everything. And, Father, while you grant me the grace to be strong and mentally sharp, help me to be aware of the people around me with dementia. Allow me to minister your grace and peace to these dear people, who are made in your image. Grant me to be sensitive to the needs of those who are daily caring for them. I pray this for the glory of the Lord Jesus. Amen

4

Social Wellness

FOCUS ON OTHERS

Do you remember Jim, the gentlemen I described in the first chapter, as being in terrific physical shape but without any friends? I suspect you thought about his situation the same way I did—"What a waste!" Jim never took advantage of the fact that we have been made for community. I learned a lot about relationships from my father. In his more active years, Dad's typical social involvement was doing things with others. The focus was not on the relationships but on the projects they were involved in. As he got older, I was impressed by how he would spend a great deal of time sitting around talking with others, not in order to accomplish things but simply to enjoy being with them. God's intent is that we enjoy other people. Our relationships may range from superficial acquaintances to close friends with whom we can share life deeply. These may be family members and other lifelong friends, or they may be recent acquaintances. The length of our friendship does not matter, but building a network of friends and having social support is essential to being well.

We Are Designed to Be People Persons

As Christians we have a good theological reason to pursue relationships with others. We worship a triune God in whose image we have been made. Long before time began, the three persons of the Godhead were in relationship with each other. Similarly, God intended us to be in relationship with himself and with others.

After he created Adam, God said, "It is not good that man should be alone" (Gen. 2:18). This applies to more than marriage. God designed all people to live in community. That is why our third approach to staying well to the glory of God is to focus on others.

Friendships with Purpose

Life is much richer, our wellness is enhanced, and we contribute more to others if we are purposeful in our relationships. Start by thinking about the benefits. What do we gain by investing in others? Here are some suggestions:

> **STRATEGY**
> Cultivate friendships.

1) We will be able to fulfill God's command: "Love your neighbor as yourself." This is repeatedly emphasized in Scripture (e.g., Lev. 19:18; Matt. 19:19; Rom. 13:9; Gal. 5:14). A friendship may start by simply spending time with someone. You may find simple and practical ways to help each other or together help others. Doing things with and for others may open the door to doing things of eternal value. Jesus said, "Do not work for the food that perishes, but for the food that endures to eternal life" (John 6:27).

2) Friends keep us busy so that we don't get bored.

3) Sharing life together can bring great joy. Friends can allow us times to laugh and have fun. "A joyful heart is good medicine" (Prov. 17:22). A number of scientific studies demonstrate the value of laughing.[1] It can be a great stress reliever.

4) Our closeness to others allows us to share not only their joys but also their pains, putting our own problems in better perspective. Paul reminds us that in the church, "if one member suffers, all suffer together; if one member is honored, all rejoice together" (1 Cor. 12:26).

5) That same chapter, 1 Corinthians 12, teaches us that within the church God has placed people with a variety of gifts that can be used to build us up. Additionally, we can learn from the life's experiences of others and from what others have learned through studying the Scriptures.

6) Our minds and often our bodies are stretched as we do things with others. Of course, that can happen in two ways. If we join others for a walk or exercise, we are being stretched in good ways. If we go out together for ice cream sundaes, it might stretch only our waistlines.

Friendships benefit not only us but also others. Jennie at eighty-four was suffering from a bad heart and could no longer cut her small plot of grass. I happened to know her younger neighbors and mentioned her need to them. Now, they happily cut her grass any time they cut their own, and she always invites them in for a sweet. They have become great friends. I also think of the ninety-year-old widow of one of my former colleagues, a trained clinical psychologist who, after her husband died, spent her days at the local free medical clinic offering to chat with patients about their emotional problems. She told me that no longer having a license to practice did not keep her from meeting people who needed a friend. These individuals have provided needed service to others while being profoundly enriched themselves.

In meeting some of the practical needs of others, we not only lift part of the burden from their families but also authenticate their value as people. No longer will they feel cast aside and un-cared for. We can also show God's love to them in tangible ways. John writes: "No one has ever seen God; if we love one another, God abides in us and his love is perfected in us" (1 John 4:12). His point is that whereas people on earth cannot actually see God, they can become aware of him by observing our loving acts. Jesus made it clear that loving service, especially among believers, should be the hallmark of Christians. He said, "A new commandment I give to you, that you love one another: just as I have loved you, you also are to love one another. By this all people will know that you are my disciples, if you have love for one another" (John 13:34–35).

Though the benefits of purposeful friendships will accrue to ourselves and to others, the ultimate reason for cultivating them is to bring glory to God. We can do this in several ways.

First, we should view our service to others as primarily to the Lord, "rendering service with a good will as to the Lord and not to man" (Eph. 6:7). Once we adopt this mind-set, it does not matter so much who we are serving or whether they deserve it. Instead, we will remember the wonderful things God has done for us when we did not deserve anything but his wrath. Similarly, we won't be motivated by what we may get in return in this life. Our motivation will be the glory God gets as a result of our service.

Second, we should make it known that we are acting in God's name. Jesus challenged us to live so that others "may see your good works and give glory to your Father who is in heaven" (Matt. 5:16). The good things we do will prompt people to give praise to God. One of the things I love to hear when I do something for another is, "I thank God for you." I thrill to think that somehow God was praised for something he enabled me to do.

Third, we can build relationships in which we share the good news about Jesus. Paul speaks of the gospel as, "the glory of Christ" (2 Cor. 4:4). Therefore when we share the gospel with others, Christ is glorified.

Fourth, we can share the wonders of God with other believers. In the context of small groups of friends, we can sing hymns proclaiming God's goodness, or, if our local church encourages such a practice, we can celebrate the Lord's Supper together. There are many ways we can worship him with others that we cannot do by ourselves.

STRATEGY

Build friendships with an eternal purpose in mind.

Strengthen Your Marriage

We need to be especially purposeful in strengthening our marriage. Some of us will approach our older years after decades of marital bliss; others will look back on years of stress; still others will find themselves in a relatively recent marriage; and many will be single, whether happily or regretfully. Each group will have unique challenges and opportunities to grow stronger.

I remember Jerrid and Linda, each in their late nineties, who came to my office after their seventy-fifth wedding anniversary. They both had health problems but were doing the best they could to support and encourage each other. I congratulated them on being faithful to their wedding vows, and they smiled, shaking their heads affirmatively. Now, I acknowledge that seventy-five years of marriage is the exception, and not many couples will see their diamond jubilee. But if we are ever so blessed, the only way it will prove to be a blessing is if we take time now to evaluate our relationship and follow some basic strategies to keep it strong.

The poet Robert Browning wrote, "Grow old along with me, the best is yet to be." Perhaps his words are a bit idealistic. Yet the astute Christian counselor Paul Tournier also wrote glowingly of marriage in later life: "Growing old together, husband and wife can come to know a love which is in a way a prefiguration of heaven, for it is less tumultuous than the love of youth, being less directed toward selfish pleasure-seeking."[2] We must remember that God uses the transparent and intimate nature of marriage to teach us what it is like to have an intimate relationship with him. He also uses it as one of his tools to transform us into the likeness of Christ. Tim Keller offers a challenging perspective on Christian marriage:

> Within the Christian vision for marriage, here's what it means to fall in love. It is to look at another person and get a glimpse of the person God is creating, and to say, "I see who God is making you, and it excites me! I want to be part of that. I want to partner with you and God in the journey you are taking to his throne. And when we get there, I will look at your magnificence and say, 'I always knew you could be like this. I got glimpses of

it on Earth, but now look at you!'" Each spouse should see the great thing that Jesus is doing in the life of their mate through the Word, the gospel. Each spouse then should give him- or herself to be a vehicle for that work and envision the day that you will stand together before God, seeing each other presented in spotless beauty and glory.[3]

There is no question that those still married as they enter old age have unique opportunities to become more like Jesus as a result of their marriage, but they face changes that might impede such growth. Changes such as retirement and declining health may lead to conflicts, some of which might be new while others stem from long-standing issues never resolved from earlier days. Dealing with these barriers to marital wellness is crucial to glorifying God. There are a number of strategies we can implement as we begin to age that will help us maintain marital wellness in our later years.

Cultivate Intimate Companionship

The fundamental nature of marriage is companionship. In Genesis 2:24 God refers to the marital bond as being "one flesh." That is not strictly a metaphor for sexual intercourse. Old Testament scholar Richard Averbeck observes:

> The point . . . is that the man will bond with the woman in permanent personal commitment that will never come apart. They become "one flesh" in the sense that they become one functional unit, dealing with life together in bond with one another."[4]

Marriage provides an opportunity to know and be known in the closest of all human relationships. In later life, with the children gone, and one or both being retired, the couple has more leisure time to be together and cultivate a greater closeness that wasn't as easily done when they were both busier. This allows for the mutual sharing of feelings and private emotions that promote intimacy. Unfortunately, some people, for various reasons, shy away from sharing their feelings. However, it's important to risk doing so. And intimate companionship can be enhanced in many other ways such as playing, working, praying, or serving together.

While having more time to be together is one of the greatest blessings of a couple's growing old, that extra time can sometimes create problems in the relationship. Couples sometimes complain of too much togetherness, which is often the case after retirement. Neither one is accustomed to both of them being around the house so much. Another drawback of too much togetherness is that it can take away one of the joys of conversation: talking about separate experiences. If you aren't doing much without your partner, you don't have much to share that is new. It helps if you can plan to have experiences without your spouse that you may later enjoy talking about together.

Dorothy and I have found Gary Chapman's description of the five love languages helpful in our relationship.[5] Chapman speaks of words of affirmation, acts of service, receiving gifts, quality time, and physical touch. It is my observation that these are not necessarily static as the years go by, and the way we experience and show love may evolve. It is critical that we be sensitive to such changes in order to continue to effectively communicate our love for our spouse.

Enjoy Physical Intimacy

Some couples in later life do not have much of a sexual relationship because it is not important to them. Provided both are satisfied, there is no problem with that. But if your sexual relationship has been a satisfying and significant part of your marriage, there are few reasons that it should not continue as you age. For those who continue to be capable of and enjoy sexual intercourse, there is no theoretical age limit when this should stop.

> **STRATEGY**
> Explore ways to increase your intimate companionship.

It can be healthy and invigorating to the spirit. In fact, there are reasons why a couple's love life may be more satisfying in their later years. These include more privacy, time, and energy to invest in this aspect of their relationship.

For those couples who are unable to have intercourse for medical reasons, there are many treatments available for both men and women. Consulting with your physician may be the first step. You want to be sure that the problem (whether a lack of sex drive or the ability to perform) is not caused by a medical condition that is correctable, including with medications (e.g., various blood pressure drugs and antidepressants). Then you may want to investigate some of the treatment options available. These decisions should be made as a couple, not just by one spouse. I have known a number of older men who have pursued hormone replacement or medications for erectile dysfunction, when their wives were quite happy without sex, resulting in more frustration than satisfaction. Even without intercourse, there are many ways to achieve satisfaction from physical intimacy. "Rejoice in the wife of your youth, a lovely deer, a graceful doe. Let her breasts fill you at all times with delight; be intoxicated always in her love" (Prov. 5:18–19).

An active marital sex life provides intimacy and pleasure as well as helping men and women cope with being tempted to have, or lust after, sex outside of marriage. These sins are not exclusive to young people. The apostle Paul counsels, "Because of the temptation to sexual immorality, each man should have his own wife and each woman her own husband. The husband should give to his wife her conjugal rights, and likewise the wife to her husband" (1 Cor. 7:2–3).

> **STRATEGY**
> Openly talk to your spouse about your level of satisfaction with your degree of physical intimacy.

Adjust to Possible Changes in Roles

A number of factors associated with aging can create upheaval in the roles that husbands and wives fill. These may show up at the time of retirement, or when one spouse becomes disabled and no longer able to fulfill his or her previous role. Many Christians have interpreted the Scriptures to indicate that the husband should lead the wife and be the primary provider. This complementarian view is the traditional one. Other sincere believers embrace identical (egalitarian) roles for husband and wife. Those who hold to the more traditional view may feel the effects of these role changes more acutely. As the primary provider, the husband might always have valued himself for being able to support his family. If that's the case, after retirement he needs to find his worth in what he can do around the house to emotionally support and practically help his wife. Generally, white-collar men adjust to helping out around the house better than blue-collar men. Working-class husbands may view their doing the house work as demeaning.

Retirement might also include a husband's trying to take over the management of the house, something he may have left to his wife during his years of employment. This can lead to no end of frustration. When role changes are forced upon us by decline in our physical or intellectual capacity, there is potential for further frustration. I have often seen a dominant spouse become debilitated and literally forced out of the driver's seat. The compromised husband or wife must now adapt to the spouse's making decisions and handling matters that he or she was accustomed

> **STRATEGY**
> Make sure you are willing to lovingly adapt to changing roles in your marriage.

to doing alone. It takes some humility and grace to accept these role changes, something pride may make difficult.

There is a crucial dynamic to a couple's dealing with any role conflicts that occur: love. Sacrificial love is the prerequisite to any successful relationship that brings glory to God. Prior to Paul's words about marriage, he makes this clear: "Be imitators of God, therefore, as dearly loved children and live a life of love, just as Christ loved us and gave himself up for us" (Eph. 5:1–2 NIV). Acting in love allows us to accommodate changing roles as the years go by. Successfully adapting to these role changes in later life, especially after retirement, may allow us to reevaluate what gives our lives worth. It is not what we accomplish for ourselves but what Christ has done for us that allows us to serve others.

Develop Your Spiritual Relationship

God is the best ally of a marriage. As my friend Charles Sell claims: "If marriage were a loaf of bread, spiritual intimacy would be the yeast." By sharing time together to worship, study the Bible, and pray, couples can encourage each other to grow in grace as well as allow the Spirit to invigorate all of life, including their marriage. Usually, life's later decades offer more leisure time to do this. Often, we think relating spiritually is sharing a devotional time, and that is often an important part. But we have many opportunities to relate to God informally and spontaneously any time and anywhere. We can intentionally insert into our daily life significant moments together with God. We have many chances to stop what we are doing and give thanks, celebrating God's goodness and grace. After watching a spectacular sunset, we can bow together and worship him as the creator of such beauty. After getting a phone call asking for prayer, we can stop and offer a prayer of intercession. If we learn from a TV broadcast of an ongoing crisis, we can pray for those involved. Isn't this what the apostle Paul had in mind when he urged us to "pray without ceasing" (1 Thess. 5:17)? Consider, too, the many opportunities daily living provides for us to learn together. All sorts of occasions may cause us to ask ourselves questions about God and His word: a sermon, a Bible study group, reading an article in a newspaper or magazine. We should cultivate the habit of talking together about these things as well as researching answers to questions that arise.

In addition to spontaneous times together with God, it helps to have formal, planned times. There is no rule that tells us how often or how long these times should be. While some couples have such "quiet times" together each day, some prefer to have them three or four times a week, permitting them on other days to have their individual times with the Lord. Couples often report that one obstacle to having devotions together is boredom. While routinely reading a passage of Scripture and then praying is profitable, I suggest you be more creative in what you do. Read aloud from a devotional book or biblical commentary and then take time to discuss it. Utilize the many helpful electronic aids that are available. Learn how to download sermons and listen to them together, but don't stop there: take notes and write down questions to discuss. Develop prayer lists together. There may be things you want to pray about every day. Lamar and Patsy have a weekly schedule: on Mondays they pray for their church group; on Tuesdays, for their friends working abroad; on Wednesdays, their political leaders, etc.

Finally learn how to serve together. Several years ago Dorothy and I realized that we had become quite proficient at doing our own things but were not doing any service together. It caused us to make some major changes. Now we do most of our spiritual service together. As we play off each other's strengths, we are learning the value of being "one flesh"—we are doing life together.

For those privileged with marriage or a close friendship in their later years, wonderful opportunities open up. Marriage should give them a taste of what their future relationship with God will be like and make them long even more for their heavenly home. But marriage, like everything else in the senior years, requires careful planning and intentional strategies.

How Can We Build Relationships?

Choose Your Living Situation Wisely

Marie was at my office talking about her loneliness. Eighty-three and widowed, she had recently moved to our area to live with her daughter and two teen-aged grandsons. The family was always busy and spent little time at

STRATEGY

Use your marriage to strengthen your relationship with God.

home with her. Though her macular degeneration kept her from driving, she could still maintain her passion for reading with the use of a special reading machine. We tried to explore ways to get her out of the house to be with people, but her living in the country and having no friends in the area made this difficult. From Marie's situation we can learn that the first thing to do if we want friends is to be where people are.

We should not make the decision about where to live based only on our current health and mobility; we should keep an eye on the future. A major consideration in choosing where to live should be the social support system we can develop for future years. Where we live will profoundly affect our relationships with others, especially family and church. I know of many retirees who have moved to warmer climates, enjoyed being there for a number of years, and then developed health problems when they were cut off from the badly needed support of family and long-term friends. They soon regretted leaving behind the community they had nurtured over the years. On retiring, Dorothy and I look forward to moving near to our children. But for that to work, we know we must make that move while we are still healthy enough to develop a strong support system that will be with us as we come to the end of life.

We need not only to be in a place where we are around people but also to be willing to invest in these relationships. This starts by using some of the increased free time we have in our older years to build close friendships. It pays to invest not only time but also money in friendships. Scriptures admonish us to show hospitality (Rom. 12:13; Heb. 13:2; 1 Pet. 4:9). Inviting friends to share a meal, sending cards, and giving gifts are all ways to nurture relationships. Proverbs tells us, "Everyone is a friend to a man who gives gifts" (19:6).

Think about Continuing to Work
Prior to retirement many of our friendships are maintained at work. Leaving a job may result in a devastating loss of our social support system. There is nothing wrong with work. I often remind people that God gave Adam a job to do before he sinned. Work was not a punishment for sin; it is what we were made for. Too many people retire far too early, which is

STRATEGY
Choose to live among friends.

especially problematic if they do not have other activities that keep them engaged with others. I hope to continue to work when I retire from my medical practice next year at sixty-six. I don't intend to work the hours or carry the responsibility that I presently do, but, God allowing, I will be happy to do something for twenty to thirty hours a week. On the job I will develop new friendships and rebuild a social network.

I am impressed with Mary Jane, who, at eighty-six, works at the local department store. She doesn't need the money, but she loves to keep busy and "go out with the girls." Then there is Ray, who, at age ninety-three, still works in his profession as a barber, cutting hair for the "good old boys." I suspect there is a lot more chatting than cutting. I think about these two and wonder whether they are so involved with others because they are healthy, or whether they are healthy because they are so involved with others. I suspect it is a circle on which one leads to the other. Continuing to work is one way to deal with the loss of relationships that so often compromise retirement. The problem is, we do not go out and get a job when we are eighty-five. If we are going to continue to work, we need to start in our sixties.

Be Involved in a Church

Within God's plan, the church should play a major role in our lives and serve as a significant avenue to our wellness, and seniors are certainly no exception. A classic text on aging and the church states: "Because of the numerous problems older people experience in our society, because of the gradual approach of death, because they have more time to think than they have had for decades previously, and for various other reasons, many people turn to religion in their old age with renewed fervor."[6]

We must not underrate the value God places on the church as the body of Christ on earth today. Paul speaks of the church, "which is [Christ's] body, the fullness of him who fills all in all" (Eph. 1:23). That statement absolutely amazes me. We, as a group of sinners being slowly transformed by the grace of God, actually represent the fullness of our creator God. One day we will be the spotless bride of Christ. Given God's view of the church, we cannot afford to ignore it. Church involvement will deepen not only our relationship with God but also relationships with his people.

STRATEGY

Consider working well into the retirement years.

Even though the future of the church is dazzling, the reality is that it can be difficult for seniors to find a church that is right for them. Too many churches fall into one of two categories: either they are made up largely of seniors and will die with their members, or they are youth-oriented and appear unwelcoming to seniors (though that appearance may not be the case).

Let us consider what an ideal church looks like. First, it has all ages worshiping God together: "Young men and maidens together, old men and children! Let them praise the name of the LORD, for his name alone is exalted; his majesty is above earth and heaven" (Ps. 148:12–13). What a beautiful picture of worship involving saints from all age groups. Churches must be intentional in developing programs to encourage cross-generational fellowship. Intra-generational fellowship will be spontaneous, but fellowship across the age lines must be planned. I have seen programs such as "Invite a Senior to Dinner" or "Adopt a Grandparent." One church I know of with a very successful small-group program requires that every small group contain at least one senior.

Even while cross-generational ministry and fellowship are important, seniors need time to be with each other. They need to share their burdens with those whose needs are similar and who can understand and support them. My wife and I are members of a vibrant church in Chicago. We love the fact that the average age is more than thirty years younger than ours. We enjoy mentoring the younger believers and allowing their energy and enthusiasm to rub off on us. Still, we need our small group, which is made of others close to our age. We get together every other week to share what is going on in our lives, discuss the Scriptures, and pray for each other.

Second, the ideal church must be sensitive to the concerns of the elderly as expressed by the psalmist: "Do not cast me off in the time of old age; forsake me not when my strength is spent" (Ps. 71:9). Some elderly with limited capacity to provide for themselves will need special help from the church. Other seniors are strong and capable, looking for ways to grow and serve. They have unique spiritual gifts and need to be encouraged to develop and practice them. The ideal church will have a ministry not only *to* the elderly but also *by* them. This can include leading congregational prayer, teaching, and, when so gifted, preaching.

Some of the contributions that seniors are particularly capable of providing are emphasized by James Houston and gerontologist Michael Parker in their book *A Vision for the Aging Church*. These include:

- Consistency in worship
- Time to devote to prayer
- Time to foster community and help others
- Demonstrating strength in the midst of suffering
- Living well in the face of death.[7]

In *Senior Adult Ministry in the 21st Century* David Gallagher adds:

- A love for children and young adults
- A respect for tradition and ability to learn from the past
- A willingness to sacrifice for a worthwhile project
- Loyalty, stability, and predictability.[8]

In addition I would add:

- A well-seasoned walk with the Lord and practical knowledge of Scripture
- Mentoring and encouraging others from their extensive life experience
- The long-range perspective that allows them to mix joy and sorrow.

There are many churches that desire to effectively mix all age groups. Pastor Greg Waybright envisions the case where "the local church is focused intentionally on building a Christ-centered intergenerational community in which all serve and are served—in which all participate according to the calling and 'gifting' by God."[9] But, even in an ideal church, seniors must make a deliberate choice to participate. For those who make that choice, faith will be an enduring journey. Many who choose not to be actively involved in a church will, by default, stagnate in their spiritual lives. They will not be stretched by the inevitable changes that come, will often become critical, and will fail to be a positive example for those who follow.

The reasons some in the older age group choose to avoid church involvement are many, but one of the most common is tension between generations. It may be caused by the music, the style of preaching, the time of the services, or any of a number of issues over which different age groups easily disagree. When faced with these differences, the deciding factor should not be what each group wants but what best facilitates the proclamation of the gospel. Paul was willing to sacrifice his preferences and affirm, "I have become all things to all people, that by all means I might save some" (1 Cor. 9:22).

In summary I quote Michael Parker: "The evidence is clear: older, community-engaged elders age more successfully and are, therefore, better equipped than uninvolved and unconnected seniors to serve God, the church, and the world."[10] The church is too important to God to allow any hindrance at any age to keep God's people from active involvement.

Develop a Closely Committed Group

In addition to attending a church that provides a large Christian community, we should develop a small group of perhaps three to five people who are committed to meeting on a regular basis to cultivate a deep level of sharing with one another. These relationships may require a great deal of time, but as we enter our senior years, we may have more time for this. As so many of my patients say when I apologize for keeping them waiting, "I have more time than money." German pastor Dietrich Bonhoeffer has a great deal to say about how to foster genuine Christian community. He starts by challenging us to be good listeners:

STRATEGY

While you are still middle-aged, settle in a church in which you can be comfortable throughout your life, continue to grow, and exercise your spiritual gifts.

> The first service that one owes to others in the fellowship consists in listening to them. Just as love to God begins with listening to His Word, so the beginning of love for the brethren is learning to

listen to them. It is God's love for us that He not only gives us His Word but also lends us His ear. So it is His work that we do for our brother when we learn to listen to him. Christians, especially ministers, so often think they must always contribute something when they are in the company of others, that this is the one service they have to render. They forget that listening can be a greater service than speaking.[11]

He goes on to challenge us to do practical things for one another:

The second service that one should perform for another in a Christian community is that of active helpfulness. This means initially, simple assistance in trifling, external matters. . . . We must be ready to allow ourselves to be interrupted by God. God will be constantly crossing our paths and canceling our plans by sending us people with claims and petitions.[12]

Third, Bonhoeffer emphasizes that we must not only do things for others but also carry the weight of the emotional burdens of our friends.[13] "Bear one another's burdens, and so fulfill the law of Christ" (Gal. 6:2). This allows us to "rejoice with those who rejoice, weep with those who weep" (Rom. 12:15).

Once we are emotionally engaged with others, we can follow his fourth suggestion and offer words of reproof and admonition from the Scriptures to others.[14] This reminds me of Proverbs 27:6, where we read, "Faithful are the wounds of a friend."

The final step to deepening the level of our fellowship is to be very honest and acknowledge our failings to others. This will lead to what Bonhoeffer refers to as a confessional group in which we allow ourselves to honestly admit our sin to one another. Bonhoeffer writes:

He who is alone with his sin is utterly alone. It may be that Christians, notwithstanding corporate worship, common prayer, and all their fellowship in service, may still be left to their loneliness. The final break-through to fellowship does not occur, because though they have fellowship with one another as believers and as devout people, they do not have fellowship as the undevout, as sinners. The pious fellowship permits no one to be a sinner. So everybody must conceal his sin from himself and from the fellowship. We dare not be sinners. Many Christians are unthinkably horrified when a real sinner is suddenly discovered among the righteous. So we remain alone with our sin, living in lies and hypocrisy. The fact is that we *are* sinners![15]

We must be intentional to develop this deep level of fellowship, and I am fully convinced it is through these deeper relationships that true wellness can be found. We may not be able to enter into such friendships once we are very old. If we want them to be in place then, we need to cultivate them soon.

Make Family a Priority

You may have heard the saying, "Be nice to your kids since they will choose your nursing home." The part about the nursing home may not be true for you, but if you are blessed with children, put a high priority on your relationship with them. As the years progress, there is frequently a migration of our closest relationships from friends to family. That is often driven by increased dependence

> STRATEGY
> Develop a small group
> of friends deeply committed
> to one another.

on family as well as the loss of friends, as some die and others move closer to their own families. For those who have a close relationship with children who do not live nearby, it may be wise to move closer to them sooner rather than later. It is not wise, however, to assume that your children will be able (or willing) to care for you in your older years. That may be especially true of a son-in-law, a daughter-in-law, or a stepchild. If you are planning for your children to be your primary caregivers in the future, discuss with them while you are still healthy all that this might entail.

Some, for various reasons, may not have children who are able to care for them, and in such cases, they may want to develop close relationships with other family members. I often see middle-aged people who are devoted to a favorite aunt. Those who are estranged from their children should seek to reconcile as soon as possible. That often requires times of mutual confession and God-enabled forgiveness. When seniors become dependent on children with whom they do not have a good relationship, the children often feel forced by guilt to help. Needless to say, that is a strain on all concerned. Some seniors do all they can to avoid being dependent on their children. If you are one of them, you should anticipate that there will come a time when you need to move to an assisted-living facility or nursing home. If you think this might be the case, you may want to review your financial situation before you stop working. It may be necessary to work for a few more years, defer your Social Security payout, or take out long-term care insurance.[16]

As you consider the importance of family, it is also wise to think about what kind of legacy you will leave your successors. I am not talking here about money but about the life's lessons that you want to pass along. I well remember my dear grandmother pounding in to me a single verse: "Those who honor me I will honor" (1 Sam. 2:30). Make sure that your descendants know the stories of God's grace in your life. If you are going to have much impact on your grandchildren or great-grandchildren, it best starts when they are young. You cannot waltz into a teenager's life as a stranger and expect to have much influence.

Dealing with Lost Relationships

A challenge to wellness in our later years is coping with the loss of family and close friends. This requires a resilience to keep going and an eye out for new opportunities to grow and contribute to others.

The loss that is likely the toughest to deal with is the death of a spouse. The way the survivor initially responds frequently sets the tone for their remaining years. Sadly for some, grief is overwhelming, and they die of a broken heart soon after their spouse is gone. We know that Christians are not to grieve as others who have no eternal hope (1 Thess. 4:13), but they still can and must grieve. Not to grieve would discredit the wonderful gift God gave of a loving spouse and deeply satisfying marriage. It is appropriate to feel the loss deeply, shed tears, and spend time remembering and honoring the deceased. In his classic book *A Grief Observed*, C. S. Lewis describes the long and terrible upheaval he experienced following the death of his wife. He referred to his "mad midnight moment." Yet having grieved, by God's grace he came though it to carry on a rich and productive ministry. Eventually, grievers will, by God's grace, spend less time grieving, reconnect with others, make new friends, and get involved in new activities that won't always remind them of the departed.

STRATEGY

Continue to build ties to family members, because later in life you may need to depend on them.

Grieving does not mean forgetting the lost loved one. As my mother was becoming increasingly demented, Dorothy and I would often sing her favorite songs with her. One day, ten years after my father's death, she started to sing on her own:

Does Jesus care when I've said "goodbye"
To the dearest on earth to me,
And my sad heart aches
Till it nearly breaks,
Is it aught to Him? Does He see?

O yes, He cares, I know He cares,
His heart is touched with my grief;
When the days are weary,

> The long nights dreary,
> I know my Savior cares.[17]

The years could not diminish the loss of her best friend of fifty-six years. She found great consolation in knowing that Jesus cared.

There are several things that can be done in advance to better face the loss of a spouse. First, you can nurture close friendships with members of your own sex. I advise married people to avoid doing all of their socializing as couples. Second, it's crucial to recognize that in God's plan, marriage is not an eternal union. Jesus made this clear when he said, "In the resurrection they neither marry nor are given in marriage" (Matt. 22:30). God's purpose for marriage is to give us a foretaste of what our deeply satisfying and eternal relationship with God will be like throughout eternity. We know this from Paul's words about marriage: "This mystery is profound, and I am saying that it refers to Christ and the church" (Eph. 5:32). In other words, he affirms not simply that the relationship between Christ and his church teaches us about marriage, but that marriage teaches us about the relationship that we have with Christ. A good marriage should lead us to love Christ more; and once our spouse is gone our love for Christ may be even greater.

A common mistake after the death of a spouse is when the survivor, overcome by loneliness, remarries too quickly, not allowing sufficient time to work through the grieving process. Though I have no research to confirm my opinion, I believe that doing this is not wise. One rule that I learned before I was married is to approach marriage from a sense of fullness, prepared to give, and not from a sense of emptiness with needs to be filled. When my wife was a teenager, her mother repeatedly told her that it is better to wish you were married than to wish you weren't. Marrying in haste for the wrong reasons does not contribute to long-term wellness.

A Richer Life in Community

As we move through life, relationships become increasingly meaningful. One of my small-group members suggests that our friendships are the only things on earth that God will allow us to take to heaven. They can be a source of joy, but also through them we can feel the sorrows of life more deeply. We err when we begin to focus on ourselves instead of focusing on others.

STRATEGY
If you are married, begin to think now about what your life will be like if your spouse dies.

Questions for Reflection and Discussion

Who would you say are your closest friends?

_____

_____

What can you do now to help others?

_____

_____

What are you looking for in a church?

_____

_____

Who would you like to see in a close accountability group?

_____

_____

How are you strengthening your marriage and family ties?

_____

_____

Where do you think you should live in your older years?

_____

_____

Prayer

Lord,

Thank you for all the people you have brought into my life. I pray that you will use them to grow me into the person you want me to be. I also pray that by your grace, you use me to help accomplish your purpose in their lives. Lead me to the right people and help me to have and share a sense of wellness with all of these friends. I pray that you will be glorified through all of my earthly relationships.

Amen

5

Financial Wellness

WORRY-FREE FINANCES

Pat retired as an executive at a major corporation when he was sixty. Well endowed with stock accrued over thirty-five years, he felt that his financial future was secure. That feeling lasted less than a year. Because of the recession and some risky investments, the value of his stocks plummeted, causing him great anxiety. When he came to my office, I asked, "Pat, how is it going?"

"As well as the stock market," he replied. He had become obsessed with his financial holdings, so much so that the last thing he did every night was check the value of his portfolio. His wife complained that this was all he talked about. Previously, their great joy had been international travel. No more! Pat said they could not afford it. Sadly, he sank into a severe depression.

Financial Contentment

As we approach our senior years, our financial situation becomes an important component of wellness; indeed, it should be. How we handle our finances is crucial to staying well. The fact that Jesus taught a lot about finances means we must follow his teaching if we are to be financially well. Jesus underscored the importance of how we manage our money when he said, "So if you have not been trustworthy in handling worldly wealth, who will trust you with true riches?" (Luke 16:11 NIV). In this passage he emphasizes how we handle our finances, for that reflects our attitude to the funds God has entrusted to us. Paul warns us of the dangers of wrong attitudes: "The love of money is a root of all kinds of evils" (1 Tim. 6:10). Loving money leads to worry, and worry and wellness are not compatible. Over and over again I have observed that the key to financial wellness is not having great wealth but having few worries. Devastating in many ways, worry will cause physical problems such as insomnia, headaches, high blood pressure, abdominal pain, and any number of other conditions. Perhaps more importantly, worry can be a spiritual problem, since by worrying we question not only God's ability to control our circumstances but also his love. This leads us to the fourth topic in staying well to the glory of God: worry-free finances.

Does having a lot of money really contribute to wellness? John D. Rockefeller was asked, "How much money is enough?" He answered, "Just a little bit more."[1] Ecclesiastes put it this way: "He who loves money will not be satisfied with money, nor he who loves wealth with his income" (5:10). More important than the amount of our savings is how content we are with what we have. Contentment, not wealth, is the best antidote to worry. Benjamin Franklin hit it on the head when he said, "Content makes poor men rich; discontent makes rich men poor."[2] Billy Graham agrees: "The happiness which brings enduring worth to life is not the superficial happiness that is dependent on circumstances. It is the happiness and contentment that fills the soul even in the midst of the most distressing of circumstances."[3] How do we find this contentment? There are really only two answers: have unlimited assets or limited desires. As Christians this is a win-win—for we can have both. Our heavenly Father provides unlimited resources, and our contentment in him will result in limited desire for other things. Hebrews sums it up well: "Keep your life free from love of money, and be content with what you have, for he has said, 'I will never leave you nor forsake you'" (Heb. 13:5). Don't miss the point here—what we are to be content with is not our savings or possessions; it is the enduring presence of God in our lives.

Reading this chapter is not intended to make you wealthy. Remember, our goal is not to be *wealthy* but to be *well*. God never promised to make us wealthy any more than he promised to make us healthy. Over the years I have seen many pray for health, when God in his greater wisdom overruled and either called them home to heaven or enriched their lives through their disease. Similarly, some in financial straits call out to God for relief, and he chooses not to provide. Has God been unfaithful? No! He has accomplished his purposes in other ways. Take my friend Pat. He may end up impoverished or even bankrupt. Has God forsaken him? No! God may know that what is good for Pat is not the financial security he so badly desires but a heart that rests in God and trusts him to do what is best. Pat can still claim Romans 8:28: "We know that for those who love God all things work together for good, for those who are called according to his purpose." Here, "good" refers to what is best in God's eyes, not what we, in our very lim-

> **STRATEGY**
>
> Manage your finances so that you do not worry about them.

ited perspective, consider good for us. How often in the Bible do we see God work out his good plans through circumstances that at the time seem very difficult? The classic example is that of Joseph, who, after being taken from his loving father, sold into slavery by his brothers, unfairly accused, and imprisoned was able to say to his repentant brothers: "As for you, you meant evil against me, but God meant it for good" (Gen. 50:20).

Make God Your Treasure

When I talk to people who do not have a personal relationship with God, I often refer to two short stories Jesus told:

> The kingdom of heaven is like treasure hidden in a field, which a man found and covered up. Then in his joy he goes and sells all that he has and buys that field. Again, the kingdom of heaven is like a merchant in search of fine pearls, who, on finding one

pearl of great value, went and sold all that he had and bought it. (Matt. 13:44–46)

The kingdom of heaven is any place where Jesus reigns. It is where he is in control, and when we decide to trust him with our lives, we are in essence saying, "I know that my greatest joy and pleasure in life will come from surrendering control to Jesus. I am willing to give up lesser things to enjoy those that are greater." This is economic wisdom. Jim Elliot, who was killed as a young man for the sake of the gospel, had it right when he said: "He is no fool who gives what he cannot keep to gain that which he cannot lose."[4]

The more we treasure God, the more we will view the things of this world from a different perspective. In 2 Corinthians 6:3–10 the apostle Paul talks about many of the difficulties he experienced. He concludes by describing himself "as sorrowful, yet always rejoicing; as poor, yet making many rich; as having nothing, yet possessing everything" (v. 10). He then states that the "everything" he possessed was because of this promise from God: "I will make my dwelling among them and walk among them, and I will be their God, and they shall be my people" (2 Cor. 6:16).

God is the greatest treasure we could ever have. When we find ourselves unhappy with our lives, it is all too often because we do not treasure him enough. We have our sights fixed on the things of this earth, failing to recognize that this world will never meet our deepest longings. If we treasure God above everything else, we will find true contentment. Learning to treasure God requires time in his presence. That will involve reading and meditating on the Scriptures and offering prayers of adoring worship. We will need to take time for quiet, perhaps in a beautiful setting, and worship God as the author of such beauty and the creator of our capacity to enjoy his artistry. As we enjoy him more, we will slowly find our attraction to some of the things in this world beginning to fade, and we will experience the joy of treasuring him above all things.

Certainly, God often blesses us with many of this world's goods. We never want to discredit his gifts to us. But at the same time, he warns us: "Take care, and be on your guard against all covetousness, for one's life does not consist in the abundance of his possessions" (Luke 12:15). Instead, Jesus taught his followers: "Seek first the kingdom of God and his righteousness, and all these things will be added to you" (Matt. 6:33). It is not that we do not appreciate "all these things," but they must not become our priority. They must not be our god. This fundamental lesson is illustrated throughout the Scriptures.

The Old Testament prophet Habakkuk wrote:

> Though the fig tree should not blossom,
>   nor fruit be on the vines,
> the produce of the olive fail
>   and the fields yield no food,
> the flock be cut off from the fold
>   and there be no herd in the stalls,
> yet I will rejoice in the LORD;
>   I will take joy in the God of my salvation. (Hab. 3:17–18)

Equally, or even more impressive, is what we read in Lamentations when the Jews were experiencing national disaster. Jerusalem, their beloved city, had been conquered, the temple destroyed, and most of her citizens either killed or taken into exile; yet the prophet could write:

> The steadfast love of the LORD never ceases;
>   his mercies never come to an end;
> they are new every morning;
>   great is your faithfulness.
> "The LORD is my portion," says my soul,
>   "therefore I will hope in him."
> The LORD is good to those who wait for him,
>   to the soul who seeks him. (Lam. 3:22–25)

Be Faithful

If God is to be glorified in our finances, we may need to redefine
our goals. If our goal is to live comfortably and have no financial
wants, we may be disappointed. Instead our goal must be to live
faithfully before God, trusting
him to determine what is best,
and allow our confidence in him
to free us from worry. Our ex-
ploration of financial wellness starts with two key principles. First,
as we have seen, we are to treasure God above everything else; and,
second, we will make faithfulness our highest priority. With these
as our foundation, we can develop further strategies for financial
wellness so that, by God's grace, there may come a time when we
will hear, "Well done, good and faithful servant. You have been
faithful over a little; I will set you over much. Enter into the joy of
your master" (Matt. 25:21).

> **STRATEGY**
> Treasure God more than
> the things of this world.

God Is Our Provider

All Things Are His

It's important to realize that all things belong to God. Therefore,
everything we have is from God. "Every good gift and every perfect
gift is from above, coming down from the Father of lights" (James
1:17). The psalmist expresses that so beautifully:

> For every beast of the forest is mine,
>   the cattle on a thousand hills.
> I know all the birds of the hills,
>   and all that moves in the field is mine.
> If I were hungry, I would not tell you,
>   for the world and its fullness are mine. (Ps. 50:10–12)

Psalm 24 says it succinctly:

> The earth is the LORD's and the fullness thereof,
>   the world and those who dwell therein. (v. 1)

He Supplies Our Needs

Out of the abundance of all that he has, God meets our needs. Abraham knew God by the Hebrew name Jehovah-Jireh ("the Lord will provide"). We would do well to think of him in the same way. He has already given us everything we have. Paul reminds us: "What do you have that you did not receive?" (1 Cor. 4:7). We are sometimes deluded into thinking that we earned our investments, our retirement plan, and our social security. How foolish! They are gifts from God.

> **STRATEGY**
> Value faithfulness over wealth.

The discourse Jesus spoke about God's meeting our needs is one of the most beautiful and oft-quoted passages in the Scriptures. Read it slowly and soak in the wonder of it:

> Therefore I tell you, do not be anxious about your life, what you will eat or what you will drink, nor about your body, what you will put on. Is not life more than food and the body more than clothing? Look at the birds of the air: they neither sow nor reap nor gather into barns, and yet your heavenly Father feeds them. Are you not of more value than they? And which of you by being anxious can add a single hour to his span of life? And why are you anxious about clothing? Consider the lilies of the field, how they grow: they neither toil nor spin, yet I tell you, even Solomon in all his glory was not arrayed like one of these. But if God so clothes the grass of the field, which today is alive and tomorrow is thrown into the oven, will he not much more clothe you, O you of little faith? Therefore do not be anxious, saying, "What shall we eat?" or "What shall we drink?" or "What shall we wear?" For the Gentiles seek after all these things, and your heavenly Father knows that you need them all. (Matt. 6:25–32)

Having provided for us in the past, we can be confident that he will provide in the future. The apostle Paul could promise: "My God will supply every need of yours according to his riches in glory in Christ Jesus" (Phil. 4:19). The key lesson here is that everything we have presently and everything we will have in the future come from him. His resources have no limit, and he will always be there. In one sense, it does not matter if we currently have it in hand or not.

He Wants Us to Trust Him

One way in which God can be glorified in our finances (and in which we can be spared much worry) is to simply trust him. No matter how many assets we have, we dare not put our trust in them but recognize they are a gift from God. We never want to trust the gift and not the giver. For many of us, God has already amply provided. But if our savings fail, or if we outlive them, we can continue to trust his bounty.

Scripture talks a lot about trust and finding our refuge in God: "Trust in him at all times, O people; pour out your heart before him; God is a refuge for us" (Ps. 62:8). When we have a need, we are invited to pour out our hearts to God and come with our requests in prayer. In doing so, we implicitly acknowledge our dependence on him, and the fact that we depend on him gives him glory.

At times we will face difficult situations in which it seems that God does not respond to our trust in him. In spite of his loving character and his abundant mercy, faithful people have been disappointed with God. When this happens we are left without answers and can only wonder. Yet even in perplexing cases, we are able to trust on a higher level. We are able to trust that he knows what is best more than we do. Too often, I confuse things and find myself trusting God to do what I want. Genuine trust, however, recognizes that he knows what is best, and I can trust his wisdom, love, and power to accomplish it. He may have lessons for me to learn that I would miss if he simply did what I desired. What he intends may be far more valuable than all the wealth on Wall Street. At times it may be hard not to question just how good or how able God is. At those times, we need to pause and think about the cross. Paul rooted his confidence in the cross, saying, "He who did not spare his own Son but gave him up for us all, how will he not also with him graciously give us all things?" (Rom. 8:32). Since God gave us the greatest possible gift when he gave us Jesus, we can be sure he will not withhold other things of lesser value. We may not experience these blessing in this life, but we can be confident that eventually God will provide.

The wonderful thing is that however great or small our assets, we can still depend on God. If in great need, we can trust him to supply. If we have all we need, we must gratefully acknowledge that it has come from him and trust him for the wisdom to manage it well and for the confidence that he will continue to provide.

God Typically Enables Us to Provide for Ourselves

Although God may provide for us directly from his own hand, he usually enables us to provide for ourselves. I love the account in John 21 where we see the risen Lord come to Galilee to meet his disciples. They had spent all night fishing and had caught nothing. Jesus, still not recognized by them, was on shore telling them to cast the net one more time; they obeyed and caught 153 large fish. After coming to the shore, they found Jesus had been cooking fish that he himself had obtained. He then asked them to bring some of their fish. Jesus then added these to his and invited them to have breakfast. All of the fish came from Jesus, some directly and some the disciples had caught through his enabling. The lesson is clear: God provides all we need; sometimes directly and other times by empowering us to do what we can.

God Expects His People to Provide for Those in Need

Volumes could be written about the way God cares for the poor. Once I heard a sermon series on God's care for the poor, based on the Minor Prophets. The speaker announced his subject and then said, "In light of this topic, I feel like a mosquito in a nudist colony." He made his point! The Old Testament contains numerous ways in which God's people were to meet the needs of the poor.

STRATEGY
Trust God daily to provide your needs, whether he does it directly or indirectly.

In the New Testament, deacons were established to supervise the distribution of supplies to those in need. The early Christian evangelists were commissioned by the church leaders to preach the gospel and to "remember the poor" (Gal. 2:10). With Paul's encouragement, Christians in Europe gave generously to support victims of a famine in Israel. The church was to take financial responsibility for widows who lacked other resources (1 Tim. 5:3, 16).

In light of that, it is imperative that God's people have a heart to provide for the poor in wise ways. Simply giving money is usually not a long-term solution; nor is it often of real help to the recipients. The old proverb is true: "Give a man a fish, and you will feed him for a day; teach him to fish, and you will feed him for life." We want to give to the poor in ways that contribute to their long-term success, always emphasizing that we are equal to them in God's eyes. Giving to the poor becomes a complicated challenge, because it is much more than simply passing out money.

Biblical Advice for Our Wealth

The apostle Paul provided special instructions for wealthy Christians. He wrote:

> As for the rich in this present age, charge them not to be haughty, nor to set their hopes on the uncertainty of riches, but on God, who richly provides us with everything to enjoy. They are to do good, to be rich in good works, to be generous and ready to share, thus storing up treasure for themselves as a good foundation for the future, so that they may take hold of that which is truly life. (1 Tim. 6:17–19).

His advice for them can be listed as follows:

- They are not to be "haughty," which literally means high-minded. They must not take credit for the wealth they have but recognize that it comes from God.
- They are not to set their hope on their riches but on God.
- They are to enjoy God's material blessings.
- They are to generously share their wealth with others.
- Their generosity will store up treasure in heaven and allow them a good life on earth.

It's a challenge to know how to apply these guidelines. Do we save for what is coming, or do we give all of our money away today and trust God to supply for the future? Do we choose not to spend anything on ourselves, or do we use some of our money to enjoy God's blessings? I know and respect many godly people who approach these dilemmas in different ways. I trust God will lead you individually, as he may not have the same plan for all of us. Approach these questions prayerfully and seek his direction for your financial planning.

Stewardship

Over and over again I have seen folks such as Pat so focused on their own needs and obsessed with the size of their nest egg that they overlooked the importance of managing it for its primary purpose: the glory of God. God is glorified not only by our praise when our needs are met and our willingness to trust him when they are not, but by our faithfully managing what is rightfully his and using it for the advance of his kingdom on earth.

Paul writes, "Moreover, it is required of stewards that they be found trustworthy" (1 Cor. 4:2). This necessitates financial planning not only for our personal benefit but for the Lord, allowing him to control all of our decisions. This approach stands in contrast to our culture's focus on personal security. God has given us much, and he expects us to take care of the things he has entrusted to us. We typically associate stewardship with the privilege of giving from our wealth to God, often by being generous with those in need. This is a valid perspective. Recall Peter's teaching: "As each has received a gift, use it to serve one another, as good stewards of God's varied grace" (1 Pet. 4:10). But that is only part of stewardship, for the term is broader than that. The original derivation of the word *steward* was "warden of the sty," the one responsible to keep pigs from escaping. Over the years the word came to refer more to a manager of an estate. He worked for the owner and was responsible to care for his things. In similar ways God appoints us as stewards to care for things that he entrusts temporarily to us and to do our best to assure that all of the wealth we have is ultimately used for his glory.

Being a good steward requires careful planning, spending, saving, and investing, as well as giving. All that becomes particularly challenging when we reach the time of life when our income begins to dwindle and we are increasingly dependent on savings.

Plan Well

One important truth is that God has a plan for us. Jeremiah wrote: "I know the plans I have for you, declares the LORD, plans for welfare and not for evil, to give you a future and a hope" (Jer. 29:11). Lest we be too rosy-eyed in hearing of God's plans for our good, we should remember that between the start of God's plan and the future hope for the Jewish nation was a tragic siege of their capitol, death for many, and, for others, deportation to Babylon.

When we start planning for our financial future, it is comforting to know that we are not responsible to ensure the outcome of our own plan; our job is to get in sync with God's plan since he already knows what is best. With that in mind we are still to do our best planning. Jesus reminds us in Luke 14:28–32 that it is unwise to undertake anything without careful planning. But even as we make our plans, it is reassuring that God can overrule them. Proverbs reminds us, "Many are the plans in the mind of a man, but it is the purpose of the LORD that will stand" (19:21). And, "The heart of man plans his way, but the LORD establishes his steps" (16:9). As we seek to determine God's plan, Scripture tells us to seek counsel: "Without counsel plans fail, but with many advisers they succeed" (Prov. 15:22). Financial planners and legal counsel are important to worry-free finances. They can be particularly helpful in minimizing the tax consequences on the estate we leave when we die.

There are two major areas where we are liable to err in our financial planning. First is underestimating how long we will live and thereby the cost of care in our later years. Do you know that the average life expectancy of an American at age sixty-five is 84.2 years?[5] The fact that you have enough interest in staying well to read this book means you will likely live longer than average. Also remember that average is only average, and many will live longer than that. The range is quite high, and many who are now sixty-five will live to be over one hundred. The second error is overestimating our future income from investments or from social security. I am amazed how many investment prospectuses are based on a totally unrealistic rate of return. These two pitfalls make planning very difficult.

As we plan, many of us should give careful thought beforehand so that we don't retire too soon. As we approach retirement, we are often at our peak salary and have a lot of valuable experience and wisdom. We have much to contribute by staying on the job. True, our energy levels may lag, and the list of things we want to accomplish outside of work may be growing. Thankfully,

> **STRATEGY**
> Take whatever time is necessary and carefully plan your financial future.

there may be options besides just full retirement. Some companies recognize the value of seniors in their workforce and allow employees to cut back to 80 percent or less or offer several months of unpaid leave each year. Such options allow us more freedom to do the things we have looked forward to in retirement yet also assure further years of income and productivity. Continuing to work after sixty-five lets us defer drawing on our social security, thereby increasing our monthly payment when we do.

Spend Prudently

Once retired we can rarely increase our savings, so it only makes sense to be more careful with our spending.

When we think about how we spend our money, we must keep two principles in mind that we have already covered. First, all of our money is the Lord's, and we must not use it selfishly. But, second, and equally true, as we saw in 1 Timothy 6:17, God delights in blessing us and wants us to enjoy his gifts. These two truths must be held in proper tension. Once our earning years come to an end, we may have time to be more careful shoppers and continue to enjoy God's material blessings. It helps to have a budget that will allow us to live within our income for many years without drawing on principal until we are a lot older. A budget not only limits how much we spend but allows us to spend up to our budget without feeling guilty. Start shopping the sales, save coupons, ask for the senior's discount, go out for lunch instead of dinner, stay with friends when you travel, and invite them to your place in return. There are all kinds of ways we can spend money more wisely when we have the time to do it. Keep in mind that how much money we spend during our retirement years will dictate how much will be left for the Lord's work upon our deaths.

How we spend money must be driven by our passion for God's glory. We need not over-spiritualize here. Remember, he "richly provides us with everything to enjoy" (1 Tim. 6:17). He is glorified when Dorothy and I give thanks after being renewed by a weekend away. One of the luxuries that I allow myself is a membership at the local health club. That allows me to be a good steward of my body and keep up my exercise when I cannot get outside. God is glorified when we buy something that makes our lives more efficient, allowing us more time to serve him. Is it possible that having a cell phone can actually glorify God? It should be our goal that everything we buy has God's glory as its ultimate purpose.

Save Purposely

It is wise to save our money. Proverbs teaches us, "Precious treasure and oil are in a wise man's dwelling, but a foolish man devours it" (21:20). We must be careful that our goal in saving is not to be wealthy in order to obtain the status and power that go with riches. Our goal is to assure that we can provide for our future needs and then, upon our death, direct our remaining savings into the work of God's kingdom. As we think about how much to save, we must be mindful of our Lord's instructions:

> Do not lay up for yourselves treasures on earth, where moth and rust destroy and where thieves break in and steal, but lay up for yourselves treasures in heaven, where neither moth nor rust destroys and where thieves do not break in and steal. For where your treasure is, there your heart will be also. (Matt. 6:19–21)

While we must take this seriously, we understand that Jesus was warning about senseless or greedy hoarding of riches. He was not forbidding setting aside funds to provide for our future care and prevent our becoming a burden to others.

Invest Carefully

God expects us to invest our savings in ways that will allow them to increase in value. Jesus told a story about three servants who were given five, two, and one talent, respectively. The first two invested wisely and were appropriately rewarded. The one who received only one talent hoarded it, not willing to assume risk, and incurred the wrath of the master (Matt. 25:14–30). At the same time, Proverbs encourages us to take a conservative approach to investment rather than taking great risk. We read: "Wealth gained hastily will dwindle, but whoever gathers little by little will increase it" (Prov. 13:11). Much of God's work has been funded by money wisely invested that earned a good return, which was then donated to the Lord.

There have been tragedies as well. Robert retired at sixty-eight from his lifelong career as a traveling salesman. He had made a number of conservative investments and was comfortable with the income they provided. All was going well till some men told him about their experience with day trading. Robert did his homework and initially took about 5 percent of his savings and started to make some trades online. Initially he did well and became more and more confident in his abilities. He started to invest a higher percentage of his savings just before the financial bubble broke. The end result was that, at seventy-two, Robert was back on the road making his sales calls, much wiser and much poorer. The temptations are all around us to make a buck quickly. The farther we are from our earning years, the more dangerous risky investments become.

Give Generously

We reviewed earlier the advice Paul gave to those with money. He teaches us "to do good, to be rich in good works, to be generous and ready to share" (1 Tim. 6:18). Generosity is encouraged throughout the Scriptures. Giving generously is the natural outgrowth of our understanding that all we have belongs to God. Paul grounds his teaching on giving on the example of the Lord Jesus when he says, "For you know the grace of our Lord Jesus Christ, that though he was rich, yet for your sake he became poor, so that you by his poverty might become rich" (2 Cor. 8:9). He concludes his discussion by lauding God's generosity to us: "Thanks be to God for his inexpressible gift!" (2 Cor. 9:15). In the same passage

Paul commended the impoverished Macedonians for giving money that they could have rightfully spent on their own needs. Paul said their generosity was prompted by the fact that "they gave themselves first to the Lord" (2 Cor. 8:5).

Since our money is not really ours, the appropriate question is not how much we should give but how much of God's wealth we should spend on ourselves. Jesus gives us two examples of managing finances. First, he commended extreme generosity:

A poor widow came and put in two small copper coins, which make a penny. And he called his disciples to him and said to them, "Truly, I say to you, this poor widow has put in more than all those who are contributing to the offering box. For they all contributed out of their abundance, but she out of her poverty has put in everything she had, all she had to live on. (Mark 12:42–44)

In the second case, he criticized selfishness:

The land of a rich man produced plentifully, and he thought to himself, "What shall I do, for I have nowhere to store my crops?" And he said, "I will do this: I will tear down my barns and build larger ones, and there I will store all my grain and my goods. And I will say to my soul, Soul, you have ample goods laid up for many years; relax, eat, drink, be merry." But God said to him, "Fool! This night your soul is required of you, and the things you have prepared, whose will they be?" So is the one who lays up treasure for himself and is not rich toward God. (Luke 12:16–21)

Pastor Brian Kluth, in his insightful book *Experience God as Your Provider*, encourages us to give both systematically and spontaneously. He stresses that there is joy in both.[6] Even in retirement it is appropriate to systematically set aside a fixed portion of our income to give to our local church. As we have additional funds available, it is also good to support a variety of Christian ministries. These may include not only those directly involved in preaching the gospel, both in our local community and abroad, but also those that minister to the needs of the poor. Proverbs tells us: "Whoever is generous to the poor lends to the LORD" (Prov. 19:17). In addition we will want to support some of the organizations that support Christian values in our culture. All of our giving should be carefully and systematically planned. Just as we seek to keep a "balanced portfolio" in our investing, we should keep a "balanced portfolio" in our giving, supporting various kinds of Christian ministries.

It is prudent to live sufficiently below our income so that when needs arise, we can spontaneously offer financial help. In the future, the government might provide less of a safety net for the poor among us. As a consequence, not only will we be responsible to provide for more of our own needs, but we will be faced with increased needs of those in our immediate communities. Our giving should initially be directed to those who are "of the household of faith" (Gal. 6:10). It is by seeing such love through our giving that the non-Christian world will recognize that we belong to Christ. "By this all people will know that you are my disciples, if you have love for one another" (John 13:35). Then our generosity should extend to those who are not Christians. As a result, some will be able to see God in action and perhaps experience his love for the first time, and our generosity becomes a wonderful investment in the kingdom of God.

An important part of our giving will be through our wills and trusts. Here we want to provide first for the legitimate needs of our families, especially those who survive us who cannot care for themselves. Second, we may want to go beyond absolute needs and provide generous gifts to encourage and help our loved ones. After that, we want to assure that the remainder of our estate benefits the kingdom of God.

The practical question retirees face is how much of their estate to give now and how much should be invested in savings to provide for their future needs, anticipating that a significant part of the remainder will go to the Lord's work upon their death. A number of Scriptures teach us to give generously now and trust the Lord for the future. "Do not lay up for yourselves treasures on earth, where moth and rust destroy and where thieves break in and steal, but lay up for yourselves treasures in heaven, where neither moth nor rust destroys and where thieves do not break in and steal. For where your treasure is, there your heart will be also" (Matt. 6:19–21).

If we give generously now, we can trust God to supply our needs (Phil 4:19). In addition to his supernatural provision, he has instituted two ways for this to happen: the family and the church. The fifth commandment, "Honor your father and your mother" (Ex. 20:12), at the least means that children are to financially provide for their aging parents, as we saw when discussing dementia. The church has been commanded to meet the financial needs of widows, though this is only to be done when the widows' families are unable to do so (1 Tim. 5: 3–16).

So, does the fact that God will provide mean we should go out and generously give all that we have now? To answer that, we must consider other Scriptures that may suggest the contrary. Paul teaches we are responsible to provide for our own needs and not depend on others. He says: "If anyone is not willing to work, let him not eat" (2 Thess. 3:10). In his parable about wise and foolish virgins, Jesus taught us the wisdom of making appropriate preparations to last till our bridegroom comes for us (Matt. 25:1–13).

Saving and giving may not be mutually exclusive. Annuities will allow us to give and save at the same time. Under such plans, we can give money now to meet specific needs and then receive some return in our later years. I know several who have purchased annuities and specified that the payments not start till they are eighty-five. They are reasonably confident that their savings will be adequate till then but are not sure they will be beyond that.

A similar arrangement can be made with our children. While they are raising and paying for the education of their own children, they may be cash strapped. Rather than inheriting some of our estate when they are sixty-five, they may need it now and may

> **STRATEGY**
>
> Prepare a conservative budget that allows you to give generously.

be willing to pay it back if we are still alive and need the funds after their cash flow improves. In entering into these agreements we, of course, must recognize the risk that, in the future, our children may not be able to return the funds or may choose not to do so.

Our generosity not only advances God's kingdom and helps others but also rewards us personally. In 2 Corinthians 9:7 Paul says, "God loves a cheerful giver." The Greek word for "cheerful" is *hilaros,* the root of our word *hilarious.* Our giving should be prompted by a joy that overflows from our hearts, but it should also promote hilarious joy within us. Later Paul spoke of "the fruit that increases to your credit" (Phil. 4:17), emphasizing the benefit to us of generous giving.

Practical Guidelines

How do we achieve worry-free financial wellness? There are several givens:

- Everything we have comes from God and belongs to him.
- He has already blessed us with significant resources, and we must be good stewards of them.
- We are able to trust him for our future needs.
- Whereas we are commanded to bear one another's burdens, we are not to burden others intentionally.
- One of God's greatest gifts to us is the ability to provide for ourselves.
- The church should help those truly in need.

Practical application of these principles includes:

- Those who are in need should not be embarrassed to request help from their local church, and the church should generously give to the poor.
- Those with modest assets should live off their income (present wages, investment income, and social security) with sufficient margin to allow for generosity and still not draw on principal till their needs get to the point where their income is no longer sufficient. Chances are, at that point, their life expectancy and, therefore, need for future funds, will be limited.
- Enjoy God's blessings but keep your present lifestyle and future plans modest in order to maximize the funds you will leave in your estate for the Lord's work.
- It is good to give as much as possible to the Lord's work. We should give generously and even sacrificially during the years that God is blessing us with regular income. In our older years, as income is reduced and the cost of future care is looming over us, it may be wise to defer giving that goes beyond that which we give regularly to our local church until our death.
- If you have more funds than you anticipate needing in your lifetime and are not skilled in investing them, give them now.
- Do your estate planning so that your funds will eventually contribute to the kingdom of God.

When we look at our global and national economies, we see an uncertain financial future. In some ways it is like the powerful enemy faced by King Jehoshaphat. To prevent worry we would do well to emulate his response: "O our God . . . we are powerless against this great horde that is coming against us. We do not know what to do, but our eyes are on you" (2 Chron. 20:12). If we keep our eyes on God, we will not destroy our financial wellness with unproductive worry.

STRATEGY

Be a good steward of what God has given you.
Plan your future finances in a way that will maximize God's glory and advance his kingdom.

Questions for Reflection and Discussion

Do you spend much time worrying about finances? Yes / No

Name one passage of Scripture that you rely on to assure you of God's loving provision for your future needs. _____

Do you have a will and trust? Yes / No

Do you need to work with a financial planner? Yes / No

Circle the ministries you currently support:

> Your local church
>
> Local evangelism
>
> International evangelism
>
> Local care for the poor
>
> International care for the poor
>
> Organizations that promote Christian values in our culture

Does your will allow for ongoing support of these ministries? Yes / No

Prayer

> Father,
> I am tempted to worry about finances. I pray that you will give me the wisdom to plan well, to be a good steward of your gracious gifts, and not to worry. At the same time, I pray that you will work in my heart by your Spirit so that I might fully trust you for my future well-being in this life and the next. Give me wisdom to know how much to spend, how much to save, and how much to give while I am still alive. Allow me to be generous with others in ways that will bring glory to you, not to me.
> Amen

6

Spiritual Wellness

PRESS ON TO THE GOAL

Reflecting on the end of his life Paul wrote, "Brothers, I do not consider that I have made it my own. But one thing I do: forgetting what lies behind and straining forward to what lies ahead, I press on toward the goal for the prize of the upward call of God in Christ Jesus" (Phil. 3:13–14). Pressing on till God calls us home—that is what promotes spiritual wellness. This has been the most exciting chapter to write, and I hope the strategies included here will be the most helpful to you. I have seen over and over again in the lives and later days of so many of my patients that those who pursue their spiritual lives vigorously have stayed well till the end, and those who did not often struggle. You will see that changes we experience near the end of life can provide us with the opportunity for spiritual growth that may have been unparalleled in our earlier days.

Where Does Spiritual Wellness Start?

One of the things that uniquely characterizes us as human beings is a capacity to have a personal relationship with God, our creator. He made us not only to live in this world but to enjoy a personal relationship with him, starting in this life and continuing on into eternity. If we are totally focused on the material things of this life and this world, we will miss out on most of what life is all about. Augustine is famous for saying: "Thou hast made us for thyself, O Lord, and our heart is restless until it finds its rest in thee."[1] How true that is. God has put within us a sense that there is something more than life on this earth. To this point, I have shared strategies with you to maintain your wellness in a number of different areas. The fact is, though, that ultimately many of these strategies will not pay off. Your body will age, you will become more forgetful, you will lose your social support, and your nest egg will get smaller. But when we consider our relationship with God, we get to the one domain of wellness that need not deteriorate over time. Our relationship with God can continue to grow no matter what is happening in the other areas of our lives. We can find God's presence and love just as invigorating on the day we die as we did on the first day we came to know him personally. It is that vibrancy and inner joy that only God can give that make for spiritual wellness, and we must pursue them with vigor.

I remember Ned, who died at fifty years of age from a devastating cancer. He had known that death was coming for almost a year. But what a year it was! He chose not to pursue chemotherapy, which surely would have been futile, and opted instead to maintain as much quality of life as he could. He was absolutely excited about the prospect of seeing Jesus face-to-face, and he shared that excitement with everyone he could. He read his Bible with renewed enthusiasm, knowing that he would soon meet the writers. His prayers often ended with "See you soon!" His faith could hardly have been more robust—an inspiration to all. Most of us surely want to come to our deaths the same way. The problem is that we rarely experience that sort of vigorous faith if we wait until just before we die to cultivate it. It comes only by living close to God long before that time. The next thing we must do as we are staying well to the glory of God is, like Ned, maintain our spiritual vigor. Where do we start?

Know God Personally

Ron, age seventy-one, was admitted to a hospital's psychiatric wing because he was severely depressed. It was brought on by his wife's unexpected announcement that she was divorcing him—after forty-eight years of marriage. Her reason? While attending a high school reunion, she renewed a romance with a man she had dated in her teens. "I want to marry him," she explained to her husband: "and in order to do that, I want out of our marriage." Hearing this, the dejected, suicidal Ron consulted with a psychiatrist who recommended the hospitalization. While being treated he was asked a rather unusual question. The doctor wanted to know if he had any spiritual resources to help him with his recovery. Ron took to heart what the doctor suggested. After being discharged, he went to church, something he hadn't done for quite awhile. There he heard that when Jesus said, "I am the way, and the truth, and the life" (John 14:6), he was claiming that people could come to know God personally through him.

Ron's experience teaches us that it's good to turn to God when we are in a crisis. It is tempting to think that if we have neglected God for most of our lives, it's not appropriate to turn to him when we are hurting. Yet God's purpose in bringing us into some of the difficulties we face may be exactly that: to pierce the deluded self-sufficiency we have clung to for so long and draw us to him. Jesus's invitation still stands: "Come to me, all who labor and are heavy laden, and I will give you rest" (Matt. 11:28).

Like Ron, all of us have offended God in many ways and have failed to live up to his divine standards. We have sinned against him. As a result we deserve his eternal punishment. In his love, however, he allowed his Son, Jesus, to leave his presence and be born into a world that would reject him. It was God's plan for him to die, not for his own faults, for he had none, but in payment for ours.

STRATEGY
Trust Christ to forgive your sins.

The fact that God raised him from the dead demonstrated that God accepted Christ's payment. Now if we are willing to confess our sins, turn from them, and trust that Jesus's death was enough to satisfy God's righteous judgment against us, our sins will be forgiven. Then God, by his Spirit, actually comes to live within us. We begin a personal relationship with him that will go on for all eternity. That is where spiritual wellness begins.

Surrender Control

From that point forward, the next step to spiritual wellness is to progressively surrender the control of our lives to God, permitting him to be our Lord. To do this we need to allow his Spirit to transform our desires and our behavior to conform more to what the Bible teaches. It requires that we turn away from the sins we enjoyed in the past, because we have found something better. As we do, we will learn to recognize the promptings of the Holy Spirit to do what is right. Surrendering to Christ's lordship is typically on-again, off-again since we frequently succumb to the temptation to regain control. Our goal should be to progressively turn over more and more control to him so that by the time we come to the end of life, he is in full control. Surrendering control is the second step we need to take in our pursuit of spiritual wellness.

> **STRATEGY**
> Allow God's Spirit to control your life.

Pursue God's Glory

Once God's Spirit lives in us, and as he is increasingly in control, our values and goals will change. We will no longer find our deepest satisfaction and joy in the things of this life. The psalmist invites us to "taste and see that the LORD is good" (Ps. 34:8). We will get a taste of what God is like and conclude: "In your presence there is fullness of joy; at your right hand are pleasures forevermore" (Ps. 16:11). As we discussed when we spoke of financial wellness, we will realize that the greatest treasure we could ever have is God himself. We will continue to enjoy the wonderful things God has given us in this life but recognize them as his gifts to us and use them to give him praise. We will also be aware that our time on earth is preparation for our eternal life in his presence. No longer will we experience our greatest thrills when people think well of us; rather, it will be when we can help them think well of God. The psalmist rightly says: "Not to us, O Lord, not to us, but to your name give glory" (Ps. 115:1). When that happens, our passion will increasingly be to glorify God. This takes us back to what we discussed in our first chapter, where we saw that true wellness is inseparably related to a passion for God's glory. Life takes on a far greater meaning because it is not all about us—it is about God; it is not all about the here and now—it is about eternity.

I know of many seniors who have avoided a destructive self-focus. I remember Jean, who at ninety-six lived in a less than ideal nursing home. Her roommate was demented and frequently cried out. Yet Jean was totally focused on the world outside herself. Not knowing what a computer or word processor was, she daily pulled out her old typewriter and wrote a note of encouragement to a missionary. I would rarely see her when she wasn't surrounded by the letters she would get in return. She loved to read portions to me. Here was one dear soul who escaped the tendency of our culture to focus on oneself and the present. She chose to focus on others and on eternity. God was glorified.

Don't get the wrong idea here. God's glory can be pursued in many different ways. It is not all about sitting in church and worshiping him while discounting the enjoyable things in this life. This morning I watched a beautiful sunrise over Lake Michigan and sat wondering why the God who designed such beauty would be willing to enjoy it with me. God was glorified. When I go out for a

STRATEGY
Develop a passion for God's glory.

run and thank God for the strength he gives me, he is glorified. When Dorothy and I are enjoying being with each other and are grateful God brought us together, he is glorified. When patients come to the office for follow-ups and report that they are feeling much better, God is glorified. Cultivating a passion for God's glory is the third foundation of true spiritual wellness.

Having a personal relationship with God, surrendering control to him, and pursuing a passion for his glory, serve as the foundation upon which we can build spiritual wellness. If we are wise, by God's help, we will do so with vigor.

Keep Growing

Our senior years can provide a uniquely rich opportunity for spiritual growth. That may come as a bit of a surprise to you, but it is true. I have seen it over and over again. Too often, we focus on the loss of our physical strength or failing mental abilities so that we don't recognize that it is precisely by means of these that we learn to depend more on God and experience him in richer and deeper ways. Recall the lesson that Paul learned in a time of great physical trial: "My grace is sufficient for you, for my power is made perfect in weakness" (2 Cor. 12:9). Perhaps you have lived life to this point thinking that spiritual wellness means only having the ability to get out and do things *for* God. Ideally you should hope to continue to enjoy and grow through being involved in God's work for many years to come. But when we are less active, when life is less pressured and hectic, we may be able to add another element to our spiritual growth. We may, for the first time in our lives, have more extended times where we can actually do what the psalmist did: "Be still, and know that I am God" (Ps. 46:10). We may grow more through unhurried time in Bible reading and prayer. In her early eighties Deb was still very active. She continued her lifetime practice of being at church every time the doors opened, helping in the nursery and doing visitation. But once her husband became quite ill, she began to spend more time than ever before at home. She increased her Bible reading and told me how much she was getting out of it since she had more time to read and think each day.

Not all Christians will experience growth like that, since having a spiritual growth spurt does not occur automatically. Like most of the strategies we are considering in this book, it must be intentional and will most likely happen only if we make changes in our spiritual lives before we consider ourselves as old.

We must remember that we can never exhaust the potential of our relationship with God. We can never say we have arrived at spiritual maturity. The psalmist writes: "For he satisfies the longing soul, and the hungry soul he fills with good things" (Ps. 107:9). As believers we can certainly find satisfaction in God, but God is such that the more we experience of him, the more we will want. In other words, we can be both satisfied and wanting more at the same time. Because of his infinite and inexhaustible nature and our finitude, both are possible. So while we are experiencing his fullness, he will expand our capacity to enjoy him and give us the desire to experience him even more. The result is that we never stop growing in our Christian life. We are not to stop in this life, and we will not stop growing through all of eternity.

Peter concludes his epistles with this exhortation: "But grow in the grace and knowledge of our Lord and Savior Jesus Christ. To him be the glory both now and to the day of eternity. Amen" (2 Pet. 3:18). We can glorify God in two key ways: by growing in grace and by growing in knowledge. It is challenging to see how the apostle puts together grace and knowledge as areas for growth. This spirals upward. The more we learn about God, the more we recognize how dependent we are on his grace; and the more he extends his grace to us, the more we can learn. We can continue to grow in knowledge, resisting the temptation to think that we have learned all there is to know about our faith through our many years of studying the Bible, listening to sermons, and the like. But, because of the depth and breadth of God, there is so much more to learn. We grow in knowledge not simply by reading the Bible and light devotional literature but by delving into more challenging articles and books that explain Scripture and teach Bible doctrine. But what is involved in growing in grace? There are several crucial aspects:

- God's grace enables us to increasingly understand our own unworthiness. As sinners we were alienated from God and, in a very real sense, dead to him. It was by grace—God's unmerited favor—that he intervened, gave us new life, and allowed us to trust him. The older we are and the more we get to know our true character, the more we realize how little we deserve God's love, and the more dependent we are on his grace.

- God's grace allows us a growing appreciation for what it cost him to bring us to himself—the death of his son, Jesus. We should reflect on the intricate series of events that he orchestrated to allow us to come to new birth and trust Christ. It is certainly "by grace you have been saved" (Eph. 2:8).

- God's grace enables us to live each day in fellowship with him and to experience his love. This often comes with a slower pace to life, which we may not experience until our older years.

- God's grace equips us with the ability to do his work in this world, as he works through us more as we age. Note how the apostle Paul believed that God's grace was active in enabling him to perform his ministry: "By the grace of God I am what I am, and his grace to me was not without effect. No, I worked harder than all of them—yet not I but the grace of God that was with me" (1 Cor. 15:10 NIV). I have seen seniors who are active and doing God's work yet are more aware of their inadequacy and fully dependent on God's help than they were in their younger years.

- God's grace is what leads us to become more gracious people ourselves. It will determine how we react toward the needy around us who do not particularly deserve our help. We may graciously respond to their needs in kind and loving ways, even at our own expense.

As we age, we can reflect on past failures and difficulties. Some of these were of our own making and taught us how sinful and foolish we were. Some were the consequences of living in a sinful world. All have been under God's sovereign control, and as we reflect on them, we continue to grow in grace and knowledge and experience more spiritual wellness.

There are several specific ways in which we must continue to grow.

STRATEGY
Determine to keep on growing through your older years.

Experience God's Love

Continuing to grow spiritually is closely associated with experiencing God's love ever more deeply. As the years of our lives go by, we have more practical experiences that teach us of God's love, and our understanding of it is based less on what we have been taught and more on what we have experienced. Paul prayed that Christians who are rooted and grounded in love "may have strength to comprehend . . . what is the breadth and length and height and depth, and to know the love of Christ that surpasses knowledge, that you may be filled with all the fullness of God" (Eph. 3:17–19). Once we feel God's love at the core of our beings, it will impact every aspect of our lives. In our older years when we may have more leisure time at our disposal, we should meditate on God's love and be "filled with all of the fullness of God." Realize that God's love is not just for today but is the basis upon which we can hope and plan for the future:

> "For the mountains may depart
>   and the hills be removed,
> but my steadfast love shall not depart from you,
>   and my covenant of peace [*shalom*] shall not be removed,"
> says the LORD, who has compassion on you. (Isa. 54:10)

Trust God Fully

In our later years, when we have experienced more of God's love and faithfulness, we are also confronted anew with our own weakness. Our bodies and our minds begin to fail, and we may have little

131

else in our lives to fall back on. Perhaps we have lived for years worshiping the idols of success, popularity, good looks, physical and mental prowess, or any of a number of others, but now they are being stripped away from us, leaving us feeling weak, dependent, and insignificant. God uses our weakness to wean us from our idols and bring us closer to him, thereby deepening our trust. Trust is essential to spiritual growth and gives us the foundation we need to successfully navigate the later years of our lives.

> **STRATEGY**
> Take time daily to reflect on and fully absorb the fact that Almighty God loves you deeply.

> When I am afraid,
>> I put my trust in you.
> In God, whose word I praise,
>> in God I trust; I shall not be afraid. (Ps. 56:3–4)

Through our trust in God, anxiety and worry will be displaced by comfort and peace.

> Even though I walk through the valley of the shadow of death,
>> I will fear no evil,
> for you are with me;
>> your rod and your staff,
>> they comfort me. (Ps. 23:4)

As we focus our minds on God, we will have peace:

> You keep him in perfect peace
>> whose mind is stayed on you,
>> because he trusts in you. (Isa. 26:3)

Be Transformed

Earlier when we were thinking about the challenges of caring for a demented patient, we looked at a passage in Isaiah:

But now, O LORD, you are our Father;
    we are the clay, and you are our potter;
    we are all the work of your hand. (Isa. 64:8)

For many years I have had an etching over my desk of the potter at his wheel—a beautiful image. I often think that being plopped down on a potter's wheel and having my rough edges knocked off would not be a very pleasant experience. Yet I can trust my

STRATEGY

No matter what happens
in your life,
determine to trust God.

heavenly Father to transform me into the person he wants me to be. Life transformation is a large part of what spiritual growth is all about.

Paul challenges us, "Do not be conformed to this world, but be transformed by the renewal of your mind" (Rom. 12:2), and he tells us that one key way in which life transformation happens is to focus on God's glory: "And we all . . . beholding the glory of the Lord, are being transformed into the same image from one degree of glory to another" (2 Cor. 3:18).

The process of life transformation, however, is often long and arduous. Our creator God knows us much more than we know ourselves. He knows what our character deficits are, and he knows how to make us into the people he wants us to be. In some ways God is like my GPS. It always knows where I am, where I am supposed to go, and the best way to get there. Even when I make a wrong turn, it still knows the best way to get me back on the road. It may not always choose the easiest road, but its computer brain chooses what is best. In a limited sense, God is like that. He has begun to transform us into the image of Christ. All those in Christ can be confident that, before the last chapter of their life is written, God will accomplish his purpose. Isn't that comforting?

We can be grateful that God will accomplish his purposes for us in his own ways, not always the ways that we may choose. I think of Mike, a retired corporate executive, who was used to barking out orders. You probably know the type. After retirement, he was not easy to live with. Then the stroke came, and Mike not only lost much of his speech but also was paralyzed on his right side, making him quite dependent on his wife. This brought a change in him. There were no more orders; instead there were polite requests. "Please" and "thank you" were readmitted to his vocabulary, and a major change was seen by all. Mike was actually happier and more at peace. Life transformation may occur in surprising ways.

At other times God transforms us in what we may consider more gentle ways. I was impressed when my musician friend, at age sixty-seven, chose to leave the career he loved to enroll in seminary so that he could spend his remaining years in pastoral ministry. He is setting himself up for life transformation in a big way.

Get Involved in a Local Church

In our discussion of social wellness, we emphasized the importance of the church, but the social benefits are only the means to the greater end of spiritual wellness. In the church we will experience the joy of corporate worship, be taught from the Scriptures, participate in the sacraments, have a sense of personal accountability, and experience the body of Christ as it functions on earth today. In the church we give and receive practical help and are stretched by others whose life's experiences have been totally different from our own. It is likely the best place for our spiritual growth.

Cultivate the Fruit of the Spirit

There are a number of character traits that God wants to develop in us. Paul carefully lists them, calling them the fruit of the Spirit: "love, joy, peace, patience, kindness, goodness, faithfulness, gentleness, self-control" (Gal. 5:22–23). These characteristics are seen in our lives as we "walk by the Spirit" (Gal. 5:16). Though God may lead us along paths that will develop these traits throughout our lives, I have observed that some frequently develop in response to changes we experience in our senior years. Take gentleness, for example. How often have I seen a stern father transformed into a gentle grandpa? Gentleness may be one of those late-blooming character traits. The same may be true of faithfulness. Many senior saints demonstrate the parallel character traits of humility and meekness to a far greater degree than they did earlier in life.

STRATEGY

Look again at the list of the fruit of the Spirit and ask yourself which ones need to be cultivated more. Then pray that the Spirit will work in you to that end.

Having made their share of mistakes, they have learned that they do not have all the answers. Even when they may have strong opinions about an issue, they recognize that there may be other valid views. Another fruit of the spirit that I often see in older people is patience. Over the years they have learned that many things take time and that it is okay to wait or move slowly. Patience is necessary for many activities that we pursue in this life, but it is also needed in our relationship with the Lord.

Practice the Spiritual Disciplines

There is another means toward spiritual growth that may be particularly relevant during the later years, when life moves at a slower pace: the practice of spiritual disciplines. These may include meditation on the Scriptures, prayer, fasting, or taking time in solitude and silence to listen to God's voice. I recently conducted a brainstorming session with a group of seniors to discuss their spiritual growth. They felt that the discipline they could practice the most was prayer. The image of the praying parent or grandparent is beautiful. One of the things that I missed most after Dad died was knowing that he was praying for me. Now, I pray for my children and grandchildren. As seniors we have time to read the Scriptures, unhurriedly meditate, journal our thoughts, and meditate on their deeper meaning. Add to this taking time to fast, denying our natural desires, and feeding on God. Reserve regular times to pull back from people and other activities so that you can be alone and quiet with God. You'll need to make an effort to develop and practice these disciplines, but the result will be an enhanced experience with God.

Get Victory over Sin

The more we grow spiritually, the less we should sin. We should follow the exhortation of Hebrews to "lay aside every weight, and sin which clings so closely, and let us run with endurance the race that is set before us" (Heb. 12:1). Some temptations to sin may be less as we grow older, but others may take their place. D. A. Carson quotes his aged father, who prays, "Oh God, save me from the sins of old men."[2]

That, of course, prompts us to ask, What are the common sins of the elderly? Ones that I have observed among seniors include self-pity, pride, stubbornness, self-centeredness, worry, unholy discontent, anger, lack of trust, and sexual preoccupations. We must respond to those sins by confession and repentance. If we acknowledge that we have done wrong (confession), the Lord promises to forgive us (1 John 1:9) on the basis of Christ's death.

We must repent of our sin. Repentance should be more than feeling sorry for what we have done; it should include taking definite steps to help assure we will not do it again. God also helps us in that. Reflect on this wonderful promise: "Now to him who is able to keep you from stumbling and to present you blameless before the presence of his glory with great joy, to the only God, our Savior, through Jesus Christ our Lord, be glory, majesty, dominion, and authority, before all time and now and forever. Amen" (Jude 24–25). God will keep us from stumbling; we don't need to pursue holiness on our own. Philippians 1:6 contains a wonderful promise for us to seize, especially in the later years of our lives: "I am sure of this, that he who began a good work in you will bring it to completion at the day of Jesus Christ."

Theologians refer to this work that God does in us to allow us to resist sin as *sanctification*. Jesus prayed for our sanctification: "Sanctify them in the truth; your word is truth" (John 17:17). Sanctification is a gradual process that will not be fully accomplished till we are in God's presence in heaven. Recall the quotation from Paul:

> Not that I have already obtained this or am already perfect, but I press on to make it my own, because Christ Jesus has made me his own. Brothers, I do not consider that I have made it my own. But one thing I do: forgetting what lies behind and straining forward to what lies ahead, I press on toward the goal for the prize of the upward call of God in Christ Jesus. (Phil. 3:12–14)

One thing that should motivate us to sin less is to reflect on the perfectly sinless character of God—his holiness. *Holy* means "set apart." It is the moral excellence of God's character that sets him totally apart from us as sinners. The longer we live, the more we can appreciate how horrible our sin is and how beautiful is God's holiness. The psalmist speaks of that beauty:

> Worship the LORD in the splendor of holiness;
>   tremble before him, all the earth! (Ps. 96:9)

> Ascribe to the LORD the glory due his name;
>   worship the LORD in the splendor of holinesss. (Ps. 29:2)

Pondering God's holiness should evoke three responses in us. First, it should make us tremble with the psalmist as we consider our failure to measure up to his standards; second, we should fall before him in humble worship; and,

STRATEGY
Frequently ask yourself,
"What sins am I giving in to now?"

third, we should aspire to live holy lives ourselves. "You shall therefore be holy, for I am holy" (Lev. 11:45).

Keep Serving

No effort to stay spiritually well can be complete without an emphasis on serving. Asked to name the greatest commandment in the law, Jesus replied: "You shall love the Lord your God with all your heart and with all your soul and with all your mind. This is the great and first commandment. And a second is like it: You shall love your neighbor as yourself" (Matt. 22:37–39). A key way to love others is to serve them. Paul links the two when he says, "Through love serve one another" (Gal. 5:13). We give tangible expression to our love for God by the way we practically serve others. Jesus said, "Truly, I say to you, as you did it to one of the least of these my brothers, you did it to me" (Matt. 25:40). Serving others is a way we can serve God and one of the most important things we can do to maintain wellness in our older years.

It was by grace that God saved us, with the intent that we be here on earth doing good. "For we are his workmanship, created in Christ Jesus for good works, which God prepared beforehand, that we should walk in them" (Eph. 2:10). In Philippians 1 Paul faces a dilemma while waiting to stand trial before Nero. Should he wish to live and continue on earth or be executed and go home to be with the Lord? His resolution was that he would hope to live if that would allow him to continue to serve others. Peter gives us an even greater challenge when he writes, "Therefore let those who suffer according to God's will entrust their souls to a faithful Creator while doing good" (1 Pet. 4:19). Even suffering is not a reason to cease doing good for others.

Our acts of kindness and their impact on others are referred to in Scripture as fruit. Our Lord taught that it is by our fruit that we will be recognized as belonging to him (Matt 7:20). James picks that up and says, "Faith apart from works is useless" (James 2:20). Our works are key ways through which God can be glorified in our lives. The Bible makes that abundantly clear: "By this my Father is glorified, that you bear much fruit" (John 15:8). Paul taught that the fruit of righteousness that comes through Christ results in the glory and praise of God (Phil. 1:11). Peter agreed: "Whoever serves, as one who serves by the strength that God supplies—in order that in everything God may be glorified through Jesus Christ. To him belong glory and dominion forever and ever. Amen" (1 Pet. 4:11).

Scripture specifically encourages the elderly to be involved in ministering to others. The apostle Paul instructs Titus to teach older men to serve as examples of godliness, and older women to be actively engaged in teaching the younger women in the church (Titus 2:2–5). The psalmist reminds us that the righteous "still bear fruit in old age" (Ps. 92:14). One way the Bible teaches the elderly to be involved is through providing a role model that encourages future generations. Psalm 145 reminds us, "One generation shall commend your works to another, and shall declare your mighty acts" (v. 4). Even more specifically the psalmist writes: "So even to old age and gray hairs, O God, do not forsake me, until I proclaim your might to another generation, your power to all those to come" (Ps. 71:18).

The ways in which we can serve are almost endless, limited only by our capacity and the needs that we see around us. Jan, at eighty-six, has a great love for children and spends time with them, taking advantage of the natural affinity that infants and toddlers have for the elderly. She is in the church nursery every week rocking the criers. She loves it, and the little ones do too. Tom retired as the executive vice president of a Fortune 500 company at sixty-five and has been spending two mornings a week driving seniors to their appointments. Joe, at eighty-six, is still quite active and involved in his senior community, volunteering with the local Meals on Wheels organization to deliver a hot meal each day to those in need, many of whom are younger than Joe. Jan and Joe are inspiring, for they are in the age group referred to as "the older of the elderly." They are doing well. But if we do not develop such attitudes and practices—as Tom is doing—well before we reach that age, we may not do them then.

There are a number of things that I have seen elderly people do better than their younger counterparts, one of which is listening. They are less likely to jump in with answers. The experience of years has made them recognize that they don't know the solution to every problem. They appreciate the value of simply offering a sympathetic ear. Several of my older friends have told me that they have more free time now for hospitality. Eighty-five-year-old Anne still drives to a nursing home where some friends are living. Unable to take them out for lunch, she brings them a home-cooked meal once a month and enjoys eating it with them.

STRATEGY

Start thinking now of ways in which you can prepare for service when you are older.

Cultivate the Gifts of the Spirit

It's not always easy to discern what ministry God is calling us to. One way to know is to recognize the unique spiritual gifts he has given us and how they have come forth at each stage of our lives. The New Testament emphasizes that every believer has been given gifts by the Holy Spirit to allow them to minister to others and to promote "the common good" (1 Cor. 12:7). Too often we consider these spiritual gifts in the context of the younger and more active folk in our churches. We must recognize that gifts are not age specific. They apply to the elderly as well as to the younger. True, our gifts may change over the years, but there is something that God will call and equip us to do even in the later stages of our lives. What God equips us to do is up to him; that we do something is up to us.

Get Involved in Mentoring

The older years can offer many ways to encourage and teach younger folk. Mentoring does not require a formal program; it often comes about through informal relationships that grow out of just doing life together. Mentoring might occur in the context of family, where the informal contact we have with our children and grandchildren may be particularly fruitful. My life was profoundly affected by the wonderful examples of godliness I saw in my parents and grandparents. Just so, Dorothy and I sense that one of our most important future roles is to impact our grandchildren.

There are also opportunities to mentor younger friends. Natural bonds tend to form with those who have experienced similar situations to our own. I have a good friend who tragically lost a three-month-old to SIDS (Sudden Infant Death Syndrome). One day she was willing to share her pain in public. Now, whenever a young couple in the church faces a similar tragedy, they make a beeline to her. My friend has learned by experience that God is faithful, and she can share practical ways to cope with the newly bereaved. I have observed that in our older years we may be more empathetic than in earlier days. We may be able to teach what it means to be "long suffering" rather than to expect immediate escape from problems. The younger generation might develop a trust in us if we are faithful to them.

There seems to be a major change in our culture's attitude toward the elderly. I finished high school in 1965. That was the era of Vietnam and flower children, when the term *generation gap* was coined. Feeling alienated from their parents, it was the exception for my peers to pursue relationships with the elderly. Today that is much less true. I am impressed by many at our church, who in their twenties and thirties desire the friendship of the gray heads in the congregation. Some in the older age group are hesitant to get involved in younger people's lives because they assume they are not welcome. That may not be the case.

Share the Gospel

The most special way we can serve others is to share the good news of God's love and his offer of forgiveness through Christ. My dad came to Christ at age nineteen, and he lived a consistent Christian life from that point forward. Dad was never backward about sharing his faith, even though he did not consider himself an evangelist. As he got older, he was much more diligent to ask those he met if they knew where they were going when they die. He so much enjoyed being able to tell them they could be sure of going to heaven if they would turn from sin and trust the Lord Jesus. In our younger years we are often more concerned about what people will think of us. As we grow older, we wake up to the fact that it is much more important what people think about Jesus.

Do What You Can

We should not be idealistic about serving others in our older years. So long as we have the strength, we should use it to the utmost while recognizing it is likely that our abilities will change and become more limited. In the future I may not be able to practice medicine, teach classes, or write, as I am

STRATEGY
Maintain a focus on serving others.

currently doing. I may become mentally or physically disabled, but by God's grace there will be some things I can still do. I frequently see my disabled patients praying for and encouraging others.

We have to recognize the possibility that dementia might compromise our ability to function. What can we do then? That is a tough question to answer. David, a friend about my age, has lived for decades with severe mental impairment as the result of an injury he received in his twenties. He functions on the level of a four-year-old. In many ways it is tragic, yet God continues to use David. Prior to his injury David loved to sing; now he sings much of the time. He loves the old Sunday school choruses he learned in his youth, singing them over and over. People often report that David's singing has spoken powerfully to some need they had at that very moment. God, by his Spirit, is still using David in spite of his disability.

Grow in Gratitude

Another essential for spiritual wellness has less to do with action than with attitude. It's crucial that we approach life with a positive mind-set. This involves maintaining an attitude of gratitude. Though we may have to face challenges that do

> **STRATEGY**
> Spend time each day thanking God for the gift of himself and other good gifts.

not prompt us to be thankful, we can be grateful for the good those challenges are accomplishing in us, and we will always have other things to be thankful for. It will all depend on what we allow our minds to dwell on: the bad that has happened or the good that is still there; what we have lost, or what we still have left. Marie has lived through many difficulties. Having lost her two children, she now takes care of her husband in the later phase of dementia, and it would seem that she has little to be thankful for. Yet when I saw a list of things for which she is grateful posted in her kitchen, I knew that she is one who chooses to dwell on the positive.

It is great to give thanks for the many things God has given to us, but the greatest reason to be thankful is that God has given us himself. Catch that in this beautiful psalm:

> Make a joyful noise to the LORD, all the earth!
>> Serve the LORD with gladness!
>> Come into his presence with singing!
> Know that the LORD, he is God!
>> It is he who made us, and we are his;
>> we are his people, and the sheep of his pasture.
> Enter his gates with thanksgiving,
>> and his courts with praise!
>> Give thanks to him; bless his name!

> For the LORD is good;
>> his steadfast love endures forever,
>> and his faithfulness to all generations. (Psalm 100)

Live in Hope

Besides being grateful for what we have experienced in the past and for what we currently enjoy, we can be thankful for the hope we have for our future. That hope can make even the most difficult of circumstances tolerable, since by it we can see beyond the present and thereby avoid discouragment. Recall Paul's words:

> Though our outer nature is wasting away, our inner nature is being renewed day by day. For this light momentary affliction is preparing for us an eternal weight of glory beyond all comparison, as we look not to the things that are seen but to the things that are unseen. For the things that are seen are transient, but the things that are unseen are eternal. (2 Cor. 4:16–18)

Spiritual wellness involves confidently waiting for our blessed hope, "the appearing of the glory of our great God and Savior Jesus Christ" (Titus 2:13). Our Lord is coming to take us to his eternal kingdom. Then "he will wipe away every tear from [our] eyes,

STRATEGY

Focus on the positive things you have now and those you anticipate for the future.

and death shall be no more, neither shall there be mourning nor crying nor pain anymore, for the former things have passed away" (Rev. 21:4). In God's eternal kingdom he will be glorified. There we will be truly well in that blessed state of experiencing all spheres of life functioning in harmony with God's ordained purpose.

Questions for Reflection and Discussion

What spiritual disciplines do you presently practice?

_____

_____

Which spiritual disciplines do you want to devote more time to in the future?

_____

_____

Which of the fruits of the Spirit are you aware that God is presently developing in you?

_____

_____

What are your spiritual gifts at this stage of life?

_____

_____

In what ways are you more tempted to sin in your older years?

_____

_____

How is God calling you to serve others today?

_____

_____

What things are you most grateful for?

_____

_____

Prayer

Dear Lord,

I was at one time dead to you because of my sin. You gave me life, showed me my sin, brought me to repentance, and led me to trust that Jesus died for me. I rejoice in your forgiveness. Now I have lived with you for some time. I do not know how many years you have for me on this earth, but while I am still here, I want to see you glorified. Work *in* me to make me into the person you want me to be. Work *through* me to impact those whose lives I touch. Keep me grateful for what I have in you and for the blessed hope that I have of being in your presence throughout eternity. Allow me to experience spiritual vigor till you take me home. I pray this for my own good and for the glory of the Lord Jesus.

Amen

7

Emotional Wellness

FEEL WELL

At the office for his annual checkup, Sid sat in the exam room waiting for me. I walked in, shook his hand, and said my typical, "Great to see you, Sid. How are you doing?" He held on to my hand and, while continuing to shake it, said, "Doctor that's your job—that's what I came to find out from you. I can only tell you how I'm feeling." Point taken! We have defined wellness as *that blessed state of experiencing all spheres of life functioning in harmony with God's ordained purpose.* Wellness by that definition is very objective, but wellness has a subjective component to it as well. We not only want to *be* well but to *feel* well. That is emotional wellness.

Emotional Wellness: Our Role

Rather than taking control of our feelings, it is all too easy to allow the circumstances of life to dictate our feelings. We may not be able to change the circumstances, but we can change our reaction to them. The Scriptures give numerous imperatives concerning emotions and emphasize that our feelings are, at least in part, our responsibility. Consider these passages: "Rejoice in the LORD, O you righteous, and give thanks to his holy name!" (Ps. 97:12); or, "Do not be anxious about anything" (Phil. 4:6). These are not suggestions, conditioned upon how things are going in our lives; they are commands. Recognizing God's sovereignty and depending on God's Spirit, who lives within us, we do have some control over

147

how we react to the challenges of life. It requires that we not only overcome being negative but also choose to think positively. Those responses will assure that in this final area where we stay well to the glory of God, we will actually feel well.

Challenges to Emotional Wellness

First, we will survey some common challenges to feeling well in life's second half.

Self-Pity

The senior years typically involve losses. While we look forward to Christ's redemption and deliverance from the presence of evil, we still live in a fallen world cursed by sin. Till our redemption is complete we will encounter disease,

> **STRATEGY**
> Take control of your emotions and choose the positive.

suffering, injustice, and death. It is natural to feel sad when we experience the emotional trauma that these difficulties create. Yet sorrow will hamper our ability to lead productive, enjoyable lives.

Self-pity may result from a number of sources. It might come from unrealistic expectations of what life should bring, too much time to think about ourselves, too high a view of our own importance, or an inability to accept change. Our world is inevitably changing. In earlier years we may have been among those who brought change. Now change is being orchestrated by those who have succeeded us, and it might not be the direction we would have chosen. Longing for the good old days is harmful and is a source of discontent that must be resisted.

It helps to realize there can be spiritual benefit in the losses we encounter. Recall the rather staggering words of the apostle, who writes: "Indeed, I count everything as loss because of the surpassing worth of knowing Christ Jesus my Lord. For his sake I have suffered the loss of all things and count them as rubbish, in order that

I may gain Christ" (Phil. 3:8). Rather than leading us to self-pity, the losses we experience should make us long more for our Savior.

Worry, Anxiety, and Fear

Worry, anxiety, and fear can be lumped together as potentially negative responses to the uncertainties that abound in our older years. There are a number of common issues that we worry about as we get older:

- What will happen to my health?
- What will happen to my spouse?
- Will I be able to keep functioning and be independent?
- Am I headed for dementia?
- Are my finances sufficient?
- Am I going to experience a lot of pain and suffering?
- Will my death be difficult?
- Will the rest of my life bring glory to God?
- Am I going to heaven?

Many of these concerns are legitimate and prompt us to make what may otherwise be difficult changes. We may resolve to adopt a healthier lifestyle or to be better stewards of our finances.

The most important fear we need to deal with is the question of our eternal destiny—heaven or hell. Jesus recognized the value of some of that fear but also pointed out the futility of others:

> I tell you, my friends, do not fear those who kill the body, and after that have nothing more that they can do. But I will warn you whom to fear: fear him who, after he has killed, has authority to cast into hell. Yes, I tell you, fear him! Are not five sparrows sold for two pennies? And not one of them is forgotten before God. Why, even the hairs of your head are all numbered. Fear not; you are of more value than many sparrows. (Luke 12:4–7)

Jesus says God's judgment is to be feared, but he also provides the remedy. The Christian message is that Jesus has already paid the penalty for our sins that would otherwise condemn us to hell. If we trust him, our sins are forgiven, and we need no longer fear. In the context of judgment, the apostle John assures us that "perfect love casts out fear" (1 John 4:18). Only God's love is perfect; his is the only love that can dispel fear of judgment. John's statement is profound. If I'd been writing that, I think I would have said that perfect trust casts out fear, and, from a human point of view, that may be true. But then the responsibility would be on us. John knew that our ability to trust would never be adequate. It is God's perfect love that allows us to trust and frees us from fear of future judgment.

While fearing certain things can be legitimate and constructive, worrying about most things is destructive. Often, we worry about matters over which we have no control. Once we have done the best we can, there is no value in worrying about our health, the possibility of dementia, losing our social support, or finances. All too often, worry about these things is associated with too high a view of ourselves, thinking we deserve to have everything go well. Worry can also represent a low view of God. If we really believe that God is loving and powerful, we should be able to trust him without fear. The writer of Hebrews quotes Psalm 118 when he says: "The Lord is my helper; I will not fear; what can man do to me?" (Heb. 13:6).

Paul provides some helpful teaching on how to handle anxiety:

> The Lord is at hand; do not be anxious about anything, but in everything by prayer and supplication with thanksgiving let your requests be made known to God. And the peace of God, which surpasses all understanding, will guard your hearts and your minds in Christ Jesus. Finally, brothers, whatever is true, whatever is honorable, whatever is just, whatever is pure, whatever is lovely, whatever is commendable, if there is any excellence, if there is anything worthy of praise, think about these things. What

you have learned and received and heard and seen in me—practice these things, and the God of peace will be with you. (Phil. 4:5–9)

Note that he makes the following points:

- The phrase "The Lord is at hand" emphasizes that Jesus will soon return for us. That should give us a new perspective on our current problems. It also underscores the fact that he is near us today.

- We should be pleading with God for his intervention in the problems we face. He may choose to resolve the situation, or he may give us peace and the ability to bear it.

- Rather than focus on the immediate problem, we should be thankful for the many ways he has helped us in the past and grateful for the hope that he will help with our present need.

- We should expect to experience his peace even though we may not understand our situation.

- Once we feel that peace, we should expect him to guard our hearts and minds to keep us from falling back into the pattern of worry.

- We need to move on from what we were worried about and focus our minds on things that are good.

- As we practice thinking about good things, we will experience not only his presence but also his peace.

It is simply a decision to put off our worry and fear as we put on a commitment to trust God's loving care for us.

Anger

Anger is not always bad. There are times when seeing injustice will produce a righteous anger in us. This should prompt us to pray, speak out, and do what we can to bring about justice. There are other times when anger is not righteous but sinful. Not infrequently we get angry when we feel threatened or when we are unable to take control of a situation, and then our anger is an expression of pride. All too often we have anger boiling up inside us and try to deny it, which can be very destructive. We need to first recognize our anger, think about what is prompting it, decide if it is righteous or sinful, and ask God to help us respond in the right way. If we decide that our anger is justified, we need to ask if our anger is directed at the right source. Our anger might be against a disease we are suffering, loved ones we depend upon, our medical team, society as a whole, or even God. But perhaps the root cause of what makes us angry is the Devil. It may be appropriate to say, "God damn you, Satan," give vent to our fury, and dispel it before it damages us.

> **STRATEGY**
> Recognize your anger, and if it is sinful, allow God to change you; if righteous, then let it prompt you to change your world.

Boredom

Because it is essential to have meaning and purpose at all stages of our lives, we can get bored when we don't have significant things to do. I love the end of Psalm 90, where Moses, in writing about the later years of life, prayed: "Let the favor of the Lord our God be upon us, and establish the work of our hands upon us; yes, establish the work of our hands!" (v. 17). Moses dreaded the thought of spending his later days doing things that would count just for this life. He wanted his efforts to be established for eternity. If we are filling our days with meaningless activities, we will soon be bored. Granted, it might be a challenge to make significant contributions in a culture that does not always value the input of the elderly, but even with limited opportunities and abilities, we can find something of value to do.

Mac and the men of his church accountability group did. All around eighty years of age, they continue to be active and relatively healthy. They are on call at the church to do all kinds of work projects. They have built wheelchair ramps, replaced leaking roofs, repaired appliances, and done many more acts of service. Elizabeth and Barbara, both in their late eighties, have found important things to do. Still able to drive, Barbara picks up Elizabeth twice a week so they can do their nursing home rounds. They have a list of fourteen residents and make it a point to see each one twice a month. Both the men's group and the ladies' are mindful of the fact that while they appear to be serving people, they are really doing it for the Lord. These folks should not be deemed exceptional. They are simply doing what they can.

Others are rather exceptional: the ninety-nine-year-old who publishes a weekly "pick you up paper" in her assisted-living facility, or the ninety-six year old who, after moving into an assisted-living facility, told me that what she was going to miss the most was "visiting the old folks at the old folks home." The point is, no matter what our physical capacities, there are always meaningful things we can do for others. I've mentioned before how we can pray and encourage others. These are activities that God can "establish" for all eternity while at the same time keep us from boredom.

Spiritual Doubt

Spiritual doubt can also be a major challenge to emotional wellness in the older years. Many of us have led pleasant lives, and some of us have never learned what it means to trust the Lord when things are not going well. Then we hit some of the hurdles of our later years, face losses, and begin to question either God's love or his power. We may not see our doubt in such clear-cut terms, but we may have a vague feeling that God is distant and uncaring. There may be no easy resolution to this feeling. What I find most helpful is to pull back and contemplate the death and resurrection of the Lord Jesus. Once I understand the depth of his love displayed at the cross and the might of his power shown at the resurrection, I am less likely to doubt his activity in my life today.

Discontent

Often manifested by grumbling and complaining, discontentment can be devastating. Typically it results from focusing too much on what we have lost (or never had) rather than on what we still have to enjoy. When we complain to others, it becomes a double whammy, because not only do we feel down but also our discontentment spreads to them. How do we deal with our grumbling? The answer is simple: recognize what we are doing, bite our tongues, and resolve to emphasize the many positive things God is doing in and around us.

> **STRATEGY**
>
> Ask yourself which of these (or others) are stumbling blocks to your emotional wellness: Is it self-pity, worry, anxiety, fear, anger, boredom, spiritual doubt, or discontent?

Depression

Gerry has been a patient for years. She was happily married to Howard, a kind, understanding, and loving man whom she cared for deeply. She has always had a melancholy disposition, but she did fine as long as Howard was around. Ten years ago God took him home, and Gerry has never recovered. She faithfully reads the Scriptures, prays, and gets out to several small-group Bible studies each week, but she is constantly plagued by severe anxiety and depression. She cannot understand why God will not deliver her from them. Gerry and I have tried every approach we can think of to treat her depression, all without success. She demonstrates just how horrible depression can be. Fortunately, I have not encountered many people like Gerry, since most with depression can be helped. But she does illustrate how challenging depression can be.

Depression is common in the elderly since losses multiply and the resources to deal with them dwindle. Of all the challenges to emotional wellness, depression is the one we need to focus on most.

Depression is most frequently characterized by a persistent sadness or anxiety that is often associated with a lack of purpose and hope. Invariably, energy levels are low. When depressed we don't enjoy activities that previously gave us pleasure, and we often pull away from people, withdrawing into ourselves. Some depressions require formal treatment, while others do not. Depression is very complicated; it demonstrates the vague line that exists between our physical brain and our nonphysical spirit. In some cases depression is rooted primarily in our brain chemistry. In other cases it is the emotional response of our spirit. The two often coexist, since dwelling long enough on negative thoughts will lead to a chemical disturbance in our brain.

Before we discuss depression further, we need to understand three states that can masquerade as depression. The first is a melancholy disposition. People who possess one consistently look at the darker side, even though they are not truly depressed. I call them the "Eeyores of life." What would the Hundred-Acre Wood be like without Eeyore? We cannot all be Piglets, Tiggers, or even Winnie-the-Pooh, can we?[1] Second, depression is not the same as grief. When we are dealing with losses such as the death or desertion of a loved one, our health, or our independence, grief is a normal, emotionally healthy response. Grieving takes time and rarely requires antidepressant medications. Finally, depression is not the same as the normal sad response to a difficult situation. For years I have been telling patients that I feel fine, but if I go home tonight and the house is burning, the kids are taking drugs, my wife has left me, and the dog bites me, I am going to feel depressed. The right response is not to take an antidepressant to make me feel good but to put out the fire, invite my wife back, discipline and seek treatment for the kids, and get rid of the dog!

The causes of depression are multiple. For some it will start as a chemical imbalance in the brain itself. This is particularly true of bipolar or manic depression. In large part, this condition is genetic. In other instances depression comes from causes outside the brain. It may start with some adverse event or pattern of wrong thinking that makes us feel down in any number of areas of our lives. It may be related to a social relationship. For example, we may feel that our spouse is being overly critical or that our children are not paying attention to our needs. Problems in the spiritual realm may give rise to depression. We may be unhappy with something we perceive that God did. In other cases depression may have a physical origin, such as lack of sleep, poor diet, or chronic pain, or it could be the side-effect of medications such as painkillers, tranquilizers, or certain blood pressure drugs. Another common cause of depression in the elderly is dementia, as we noted earlier. In such cases, depression might be one of the earlier signs.

Depression frequently starts in the emotional realm when, for example, we become overstressed and succumb to anxiety. Whether the depression is initiated in social, spiritual, physical, or emotional realms, it may lead to inappropriate behaviors that make us feel sadder and create a downward spiral. Eventually it leads to a chemical imbalance in the emotional centers of our brain and to true clinical depression. In that state, the brain simply does not work as it normally would, and treatment is necessary.

The treatments for depression are as varied as the causes. In the case of bipolar depression, where the problem is often genetic and starts in the brain chemistry, long-term use of medication is typically required. When dealing with depression triggered by external circumstances, it is most helpful to seek professional (possibly pastoral) counseling to explore the root cause of the depression and deal with it directly. This can be difficult to do since depression robs us of the energy and insight necessary to carefully think through the situation. If the root cause is interpersonal, it may help to have a counselor mediate an intervention between the parties involved. When the root cause is an improper understanding of God, his love, or his forgiveness, solid biblical teaching may be the answer. At times, however, the depression itself can interfere with the insight necessary to assess the underlying cause. In those cases, it is helpful to artificially stimulate the deficient brain chemicals to allow for clearer thinking. This is most commonly done by the use of antidepressant medications. They are frequently effective but rarely should be viewed as the ultimate cure. It must be remembered that they only make us feel good; they do not correct the underlying problem. Once they become effective and the depression begins to lift, counseling may be more effective.

As alternatives to medication it has been shown that exercise, to the tune of a thirty-minute walk each day, can be significantly beneficial. For those who suffer from depression that interferes with sleep, doing something that allows restful sleep can help. We should never forget the value of uplifting friendships when we are feeling depressed. I was taught once to categorize my relationships from the VDPs (very draining people) all the way to the VIPs (very invigorating people) and to make sure that if I spend time with a VDP, I schedule equal time with a VIP. It makes sense. When dealing with depression in the very elderly, especially when associated with dementia, it is rarely possible to get to the root cause. In those situations, long-term use of an antidepressant is typically safe and effective.

Depression may also have a positive result, for God might use it to accomplish his purposes in our lives. When going through a season of depression we should ask what God's purpose is. Biebel and Koenig write:

> God has a purpose in all that he causes or allows. In other words, he is going somewhere in our lives. The question is: Are we willing to go there too—on his terms, not ours? Whatever it takes, even depression? Surely, the mere consideration of these questions is not a waste of time. Their resolution is, for many, the pathway to purpose and fulfillment, even joy.[2]

The great preacher Charles Spurgeon is said to have spent an average of a week each month in bed, unable to get up because of his depression. He wrote, however, that God used his depression to develop his humility, give power to his ministry, and prepare him for spiritual victories.[3] Martin Luther was not infrequently severely depressed. He wrote that his depression drove him back to the Scriptures, the sacraments, and the fellowship of the church.[4]

Consider how many of the psalms were written out of the depths of depression, often when the psalmist felt deserted by God. David had great insight when he wrote:

> How long, O Lord? Will you forget me forever?
>> How long will you hide your face from me?
> How long must I take counsel in my soul
>> and have sorrow in my heart all the day?
> How long shall my enemy be exalted over me?
> Consider and answer me, O Lord my God;
>> light up my eyes, lest I sleep the sleep of death. (Ps. 13:1–3)

While David was crying out for God's presence, he recognized that what needed changing was not God; David needed to see what was really going on. Depression is not always a sign of spiritual or emotional weakness; it may be an indication that God has chosen to enrich our lives through it. Depression will often increase our dependence on God and allow us to see our own lives, as well as the needs of others, in proper perspective.

STRATEGY

If you recognize that you are depressed, cry out to God and take appropriate steps to deal with it.

In sum, depression is not always a barrier to emotional wellness; by God's grace, it may be a means to it. It therefore serves as a segue to considering ways to emotional wellness.

Ways to Emotional Wellness

Feel the Emotions of Life Deeply

Before we think about positive emotions, we must recognize the risk of having no emotional response at all and taking an "I don't care anymore" attitude. Over the years I have seen too many people do that. For them, life loses much of its meaning. As we age, we need to make it one of our goals to feel our emotions more deeply and allow them to drive us to action. I was disappointed when I asked Charlie to help with his grandson's drinking problem, since I thought Charlie might be the one person who could help. Instead he said, "I'm sorry, but he has made his own choices, and I am not going to interfere." Charlie basically said, "I don't care."

In our later years there is a temptation to feel the emotions of life less deeply. I suspect it is a means to protect ourselves from being hurt when losses come. Yet the Scriptures teach us to "rejoice with those who rejoice, weep with those who weep" (Rom. 12:15). The great Puritan theologian Jonathan Edwards wrote:

> That religion which God requires, and will accept, does not consist in weak, dull, and lifeless wishes, raising us but a little above a state of indifference: God, in his word, greatly insists upon it, that we be . . . "fervent in spirit," and our hearts be vigorously engaged.[5]

If we are going to respond fervently, let us consider some of the ways.

Joy

"Rejoice in the Lord always; again I will say, rejoice" (Phil. 4:4). So wrote the imprisoned apostle as he sat under house arrest chained to a Roman guard. He was speaking not of a joy prompted by happy circumstances but of a joy,

STRATEGY
Determine to feel the emotions of life deeply within your soul.

rooted in the Lord, capable of buoying him over tough situations.

159

Wellness for the Glory of God

This is one of those imperatives we discussed earlier. He is literally commanding his readers to be joyful. All too often we allow our circumstances to determine how we feel. But in circumstances that may not be all that joyful, we can still determine to have joy, and this does not have to be exclusively an inward joy. It often helps to get together with others and have a good laugh. There is still such a thing as good, clean humor, and a hearty belly laugh is good for the soul. I have a couple of patients who never come to the office without a joke to tell me or a comic strip to share. I typically find these jokes delightful; not only do they make me laugh, but the patients get a real kick out of sharing them. "A joyful heart is good medicine, but a crushed spirit dries up the bones" (Prov. 17:22).

Love

Loving others and, in turn, feeling their love play a major role in being emotionally healthy. Doing this can become difficult as the years go by and we outlive or become separated from many of our closest friends. That is when it is critical to have loving relationships with younger people. Most likely, these will be family members, but not exclusively. I remember Judy, who at eighty-nine was disabled with arthritis and emphysema. Carol, a good friend of Judy's in her early fifties, was devoted to her. She would bring her to the office, go over all of her medications, and make sure everything was just right. After the office visit, they would go out for lunch together. Carol was an invaluable help to Judy during her final months. Similarly, Judy's uplifting spirit was an encouragement to Carol. I have seen too many over the years who say, "There is no one left who loves me." The only response to that dilemma is to find someone new to love.

Gratitude

We have already discussed gratitude as an essential part of spiritual wellness, but we also need to mention the key role it plays in staying emotionally healthy. Reviewing, with thanksgiving, the many ways God has blessed will not only please God; it will lift our spirits.

> Count your blessings, name them one by one,
> Count your blessings, see what God hath done!
> Count your blessings, name them one by one,
> And it will surprise you what the Lord hath done.[6]

Get Excited

You may be thinking, *What? Getting excited is not a typical emotional response to the challenges of aging.* True, it isn't; but it is a healthy response. Don't just sit there. Do something. If you begin to feel sorry for yourself, find others who are worse off and get excited about helping them. If you feel angry about the direction the local authorities are going, talk to them or write a letter.

STRATEGY

Consider what you need to do to develop positive emotional traits.

Taking positive action is a wonderful way to keep emotionally well. Do it carefully, taking time to ask for God's direction and help as well as getting the counsel of others. But then do something. Our emotions too often determine how we spend our time. Let us not forget that how we spend our time can set the tone of our emotions.

Deal Well with Losses

Since getting older includes facing losses, we must learn how to respond to them. There are basically three options. We can allow losses to defeat us, we can deny them, or we can accept them. For emotional wellness we must grieve appropriately but then pick up and go forward. Stephen Sapp gives wise advice:

> Christians do not need to deny the very real losses involved in growing older. Throughout its history, Christianity has insisted that the suffering of Jesus was totally real. Indeed, the denial of

the reality of Jesus' suffering—the Docetic claim that he only *seemed* to suffer and to die—was explicitly condemned as one of the most dangerous of the early heresies that threatened Christianity. No, Christians acknowledge the reality and pain of their losses, and the reality and pain become marks of identification with Christ and a sign of communion with him as a true disciple.[7]

Rather than deny losses, we face them by crying out to God, freely telling him how we feel. There are many biblical examples of this:

O Lord, all my longing is before you;
    my sighing is not hidden from you.
My heart throbs; my strength fails me,
    and the light of my eyes—it also has gone from me.
        (Ps. 38:9–10)

Do not forsake me, O LORD!
    O my God, be not far from me!
Make haste to help me,
    O Lord, my salvation! (Ps. 38:21–22)

Awake! Why are you sleeping, O Lord?
    Rouse yourself! Do not reject us forever!
Why do you hide your face?
    Why do you forget our affliction and oppression?
For our soul is bowed down to the dust;
    our belly clings to the ground.
Rise up; come to our help!
    Redeem us for the sake of your steadfast love! (Ps. 44:23–26)

We acknowledge our feelings, allowing them to penetrate deeply into our souls. We cry out to God in our pain as we shed real tears. There is no sense in pretending that we have not been hurt. God well knows our thoughts. "But you, O LORD, know me; you see me, and test my heart" (Jer. 12:3).

I recall Midge, who was frequently in the office with excruciating headaches, which never responded to medications. One day the headache caused such intense nausea and vomiting that she became dehydrated. She required hospitalization to receive intravenous fluids. When I saw her that first night at the hospital, I asked, "Midge, is there anything in your life that you never told me about?" She then started to cry as she told me a horrible experience of abuse she had endured in grade school. She then continued to cry through the entire night. When I saw her the next morning, the headache was gone. I suggested that perhaps the headache was due to the pressure of all those stored-up tears. Her headache never came back. Appropriate grief allows us to deal with losses well and is essential to emotional wellness.

Resilience

After we have cried out from our hearts to God in response to our losses, we must ask him to enable us to move on. "Weeping may tarry for the night, but joy comes with the morning" (Ps. 30:5). This ability to start afresh is critical to overcoming grief and depression.

Candace was an effervescent eighty-six-year-old. Married young, she had four children before she was twenty-five. Later, after her husband was tragically killed, she successfully raised the youngsters on her own. After they were grown, she fell in love with her husband's former business partner. They married and together rehabbed an old Victorian home near his alma mater. He then died, and she filled the house with international students studying music. She loved being the students' cheerleader and guide to American culture. They introduced her to the music world of the university. Their concerts and recitals energized her. After she told me her story, I declared, "What an amazing life!" Her retort was, "No, I have had five amazing lives: one as a single, one as a married mother, one as a single parent, one as a married grandmother, and now in the boarding house—and I enjoyed every one." Now that is resilience if I have ever seen it. Candace is one of those dynamic women who is always out to make the best of every situation. She was not blessed with an easy life, nor was her resilience programmed into her genes. She deliberately chose to make the most of every situation by deciding to keep looking forward and refusing to be put down by the struggles of the past. Facing her losses, she grieved appropriately and determined to pick up from there. Life for Candace was like playing a card game, and she was determined to play every hand as best she could.

The problem is that we are not all Candaces. Some of our losses may seem bigger than we are. Resilience may be easier to write or talk about than to practice. It frequently requires resources from outside ourselves, such as support from family or friends. Ultimately all of our resources come from our Lord. I have consistently seen my patients emboldened by him. "God is our refuge and strength, a very present help in trouble" (Ps. 46:1). If we are to receive God's help, we will need to appropriate Paul's prayer for ourselves: "May you be strengthened with all power, according to his glorious might, for all endurance and patience with joy" (Col. 1:12).

> **STRATEGY**
> When faced with losses, allow time to grieve and then pick up and move on.

Contentment

Doris, age ninety-two, is one of my most delightful patients. Widowed at eighty-five after sixty-five years of a wonderful marriage, she now lives with her daughter. Though she is somewhat forgetful, she never fails to tell me how blessed she is to have her daughter and feel so well loved. Being slowed down by severe arthritis has not dampened her spirit. Never complaining, she is always radiating a sense of contentment, which is the key factor in her emotional wellness. In talking to Doris I found two major factors that contribute to her contentment. First, she deliberately chooses not to focus on what she has lost but rather on what she still has.

Second, she has no delusions as to what her life should be like at this stage; her expectations are much more realistic than many others I have known.

If we are going to experience contentment, we must first understand that it has three essential tenses: peace with our past, satisfaction in the present, and confidence for the future.

We start with being at peace with our past. If we look backward, always wishing our lives had been better, we are constantly sowing the seeds of discontent in the present. To avoid this, we must believe that God has had a specific purpose for every stage of our lives. Realizing that his purposes have been accomplished, we can move contentedly into the future. But contentment also depends on our coming to peace with our sin and failures. Even these need not rob us of contentment, since God offers us forgiveness through Christ. Once we have experienced his forgiveness, we need not allow a spoiled conscience to breed discontent.

To achieve contentment we must also be satisfied with our present life. Some of this will come from applying principles developed in our earlier chapters. Those principles are worth repeating here:

- Do your best to preserve your physical health and keep active, even when you have physical limitations.
- Enjoy mental activities to keep your mind sharp.
- Develop fulfilling relationships, being sure to cultivate new friendships with people you find invigorating, especially those who are younger than you.
- Plan your finances so that you do not worry about them.
- Find your greatest joy and satisfaction in God.

In each of these domains of wellness, we are challenged to take charge and do our best. The end result will lead to some degree of satisfaction. No matter how hard we try to be healthy in each domain of life, the reality is that in most of these areas, the wellness we have achieved will eventually be depleted. Our physical health or our mind may fail, we might lose much of our social support, or our finances will dwindle. The only area that need not fail is the satisfaction we receive from our relationship with God. If we enjoy a daily, personal relationship with him and have grown in our appreciation of his love, satisfaction from him will compensate for many of the losses we experience in other domains of wellness.

I have met scores of elderly patients who have found this to be true in their lives. Psalm 73 is a favorite of many of them: "Whom have I in heaven but you? And there is nothing on earth that I desire besides you" (v. 25). The apostle Paul exemplified this amazing attitude. He wrote, "Not that I am speaking of being in need, for I have learned in whatever situation I am to be content" (Phil. 4:11). He did not need much; food and clothing were enough (1 Tim 6:8). Even in the midst of extreme hardship, Paul was satisfied with what he had. "For the sake of Christ, then, I am content with weaknesses, insults, hardships, persecutions, and calamities. For when I am weak, then I am strong" (2 Cor. 12:10). Paul did not say that he enjoyed difficult circumstances, but that he was content in the midst of them. The presence of God's Spirit in our lives today allows many of the other things that would compete for our affections to be less attractive, permitting us to be satisfied without them. As we draw closer to our heavenly home, our walk with the Lord is vital. Our spiritual wellness begins to overpower the impact of the losses we have in other spheres. We can still be satisfied.

Experiencing contentment also requires facing the future with confidence. God's promises, such as this one, can put us at ease:

> When you pass through the waters, I will be with you;
>   and through the rivers, they shall not overwhelm you;
> when you walk through fire you shall not be burned,
>   and the flame shall not consume you.
> For I am the LORD your God,
>   the Holy One of Israel, your Savior. . . .

Because you are precious in my eyes,
and honored, and I love you. . . .
Fear not, for I am with you. (Isa. 43:2–5)

The long-term future that we anticipate as Christians is amazing: "What no eye has seen, nor ear heard, nor the heart of man imagined, what God has prepared for those who love him" (1 Cor. 2:9). There is a bit of a paradox here. As we long for something far better, we find ourselves more patient and content with things as they are. Puritan Jeremiah Burroughs writes, "You never learned the mystery of contentment unless it may be said of you that, just as you are the most contented man, so you are also the most unsatisfied man in the world."[8] We identify with David when he writes, "As for me, I shall behold your face in righteousness; when I awake, I shall be satisfied with your likeness" (Ps. 17:15). Until we are in God's presence, we know we will not be fully satisfied, but by knowing what our future holds, we can be content in the present. We understand that what we have down here is like a down payment on our eventual inheritance (Eph.

> **STRATEGY**
> Follow Paul's example:
> "I have learned in whatever situation I am to be content"
> (Phil. 4:11).

1:14). We do not expect life on this earth to rival what we will have in heaven, and in that hope we can endure patiently and feel well.

Feeling Well

You will remember Henry, whom we met in the preface. At ninety-five he comes in to the office with his walker and responds to my asking "How is it going, my friend?" by smiling, giving me a strong handshake, and saying, "Praise the Lord, I'm well, thank you!" I believe Henry means that he *is* well, but I also suspect that he *feels* well. No question that his heart is weak and causes him shortness of breath, but mentally he is pretty sharp.

After losing his wife, he moved into a retirement community where he made many friends, but then his funds ran out, so last year he moved in with his daughter, who was seventy and had recently lost her husband. To this day they enjoy each other's company, and his social security helps with their finances. He is still able to go to church and makes it a point to say something encouraging to everyone he sees. That makes him a favorite of many in the congregation. His eyes are not good enough to read much, but he enjoys listening to Christian radio, and his daughter supplies him with books on tape that keep his mind occupied. At other times he sits quietly, dozing on and off, but when alert he is conscious of the Lord's presence. He often sings one of the hymns he loves or quotes some of his favorite Scripture passages to himself. His days go by without much change, but he is blissfully content.

Henry knows that God has always been in control of his life and is confident that he still is. He is not plagued by his past failures, knowing they have been forgiven. He recognizes that God has a purpose for his life each day, and even with his current limitations he knows he can bring glory to God. He finds great hope anticipating his eternal future with God. In sum, Henry has chosen to make God the unifying focus of his life, and he experiences *shalom*—he is at peace even though some areas of his life are not as he might have wished. He has learned to place more value on spiritual realities than on his physical, mental, social, or financial wellness, and on that basis he feels well.

Henry is one of my heroes. I am sixty-five. Ninety-five seems far into the future, but if God wills, I want to be as well as possible thirty years from now. If that is going to be the case, I need to make some deliberate changes in my life—*now*! I suspect you do too. I pray God's blessing as you experience wellness for the glory of God.

Questions for Reflection and Discussion

1) Rate how you are doing on the following challenges to emotional wellness:

Self-pity

    Major problem 1 2 3 4 5 6 7 8 9 10 No problem

Worry, anxiety, and fear

    Major problem 1 2 3 4 5 6 7 8 9 10 No problem

What do you worry about?

_____

_____

_____

Anger

    Major problem 1 2 3 4 5 6 7 8 9 10 No problem

Boredom

    Major problem 1 2 3 4 5 6 7 8 9 10 No problem

Doubt

    Major problem 1 2 3 4 5 6 7 8 9 10 No problem

Discontentment

    Major problem 1 2 3 4 5 6 7 8 9 10 No problem

Depression

    Major problem 1 2 3 4 5 6 7 8 9 10 No problem

2) Now rate how you are faring in the positive ways to emotional wellness:

Joy

    Very low 1 2 3 4 5 6 7 8 9 10 Very high

Love

Very low   1   2   3   4   5   6   7   8   9   10   Very high

Gratitude

Very low   1   2   3   4   5   6   7   8   9   10   Very high

Excitement

Very low   1   2   3   4   5   6   7   8   9   10   Very high

Dealing well with losses

Very low   1   2   3   4   5   6   7   8   9   10   Very high

Resilience

Very low   1   2   3   4   5   6   7   8   9   10   Very high

Contentment

Very low   1   2   3   4   5   6   7   8   9   10   Very high

3) What can you do to improve any areas that you ranked less than 5.

_____

_____

_____

_____

Prayer

Gracious Father,

It may sound ridiculous, but I would love to be truly well on the day I die. I thank you for allowing me to know you through the Lord Jesus and for the expectation I have of being with you in heaven for all eternity. Grant me the wisdom and strength to make the changes I need to make in each domain of life to be well to your glory. I pray that you will let me experience your love and your presence in such a way that they become the foundation of my wellness. Do not let me pursue the things of this earth that will not ultimately satisfy, but allow me to pursue you and your glory. I long for the day when I will no longer be tempted by lesser things but when, in your presence, I will be able to share in your glory and find my heart fully satisfied. Thank you for the hope I have in Jesus.

Amen

Conclusion

PUTTING IT ALL TOGETHER

Below and on the following pages write down the changes that you need to make in your life. Include the steps you need to take to make them and a date by which you will commit to get started.

Change   Date

Change   Date

Change   Date

Change   Date

Notes

Chapter 1: What Is Wellness?

1. Motivational Quotes.com, http://www.motivatingquotes.com/goalsq.htm (accessed October 27, 2011).
2. Johannes Pedersen, *Israel, Its Life and Culture* (London: Oxford University Press, 1959), 263.
3. I am deeply indebted in this whole section to the works of John Piper and Jonathan Edwards, who have written so profoundly on our pursuit of God's glory. In particular I would refer you to Jonathan Edwards, "The End for Which God Created the World" in John Piper's, *God's Passion for His Glory* (Wheaton, IL: Crossway, 1998), 125–251.

Chapter 2: Physical Wellness

1. Richard Train, "Sarcopenia: As We Age Muscle Loss Occurs," http://ezinearticles.com/? Sarcopenia:-As-We-Age-Muscle-Loss-Occurs&id=297128 (accessed May 26, 2009).
2. Ibid.
3. The Center for Disease Control has a wonderful website that is helpful for understanding the principles of diet and exercise. Most of the suggestions I make in this chapter fall in line with their recommendations. https://www.google.com/search?sourceid=ie7&q= CDC+health+diet&rls=com.microsoft:en-us:IE-Address&ie=UTF-8&oe=UTF-8&rlz =1I7TSHB_enUS334US334.
4. As an example, after several small studies looking at the relationship of vitamin E to prostate cancer, there was no clear consensus. A large, well-designed study was published in October 2011 that demonstrated rather convincingly that taking vitamin E actually increased the risk of prostate cancer by 17 percent. What has been felt by many to be a harmless and hopefully helpful supplement was never proved to be helpful, and now there is strong evidence that it is harmful. Eric Klein, et al., *Journal of the American Medical Association* 306 (October 2011): 1549–56.

Chapter 3: Mental Wellness

1. One excellent resource that follows this plan to allow you to read through the Old Testament once and the New Testament and Psalms twice over two years, and adds an excellent devotional commentary, is the two-volume set by D. A. Carson, *For the Love of God: A Daily Companion for Discovering the Riches of God's Word* (Wheaton, IL: Crossway, 1998).
2. John Piper has developed these thoughts further in his book *Think: The Life of the Mind and the Love of God* (Wheaton, IL: Crossway, 2010).
3. Nicola T. Lautenschlager, et al., "Effect of Physical Activity on Cognitive Function in Older Adults at Risk for Alzheimer Disease: A Randomized Trial," *Journal of the American Medical Association* 300 (2008): 1027–37.
4. Jean Léonie Bergeron, et al., "Cognitive Intervention Programs for Individuals with Mild Cognitive Impairment: Systematic Review of the Literature," *American Journal of Geriatric Psychiatry* 18 (April 2010): 281–96.

5. http://summaries.cochrane.org/search/site?f[0]=im_field_stage%3A3&f[1]=im_field _terms_archie_topics%3A1198&f[2]=im_field_terms_archie_topics%3A1588 (accessed May 21, 2013).

6. B. K. Windblad, et al., "Mild Cognitive Impairment—beyond Controversies, towards a Consensus," International Working Group on Mild Cognitive Impairment," *Journal of Internal Medicine* 256 (September 2004): 240–46.

7. Ronald E. Clements, *Exodus*, Cambridge Bible Commentary on The New English Bible (London: Cambridge University Press, 1972), 125.

8. R. Kent Hughes, *Disciplines of a Godly Man* (Wheaton, IL: Crossway, 2001), 34.

9. Peter Rabins and Nancy Mace, *The 36-Hour Day: A Family Guide to Caring for People with Alzheimer Disease, Related Dementing Illnesses, and Memory Loss* (New York: Warner, 2006).

10. http://summaries.cochrane.org/search/site?f[0]=im_field_stage%3A3&f[1]]=im_field _archie_topics%3A1198&f[2]]=im_field_terms_archie_topics%3A1588 (accessed May 10, 2012).

11. John Dunlop, *Finishing Well to the Glory of God: Strategies from a Christian Physician* (Wheaton, IL: Crossway, 2011), 197–98.

Chapter 4: Social Wellness

1. Mark Stibich, "Laughter Extends Life," http://longevity.about.com/b/2007/03/28 /laughter-extends-life.htm (accessed June 23, 2012).

2. Paul Tournier, *Learn to Grow Old*, trans. Edwin Hudson (New York: Harper & Row, 1972), 94.

3. Tim Keller, *The Meaning of Marriage: Facing the Complexities of Commitment with the Wisdom of God* (New York: Dutton, 2011), 121.

4. Richard Averbeck, "Wisdom from the Old Testament," in *Why the Church Needs Bio-ethics: A Guide to Wise Engagement with Life's Challenges*, ed. John F. Kilner (Grand Rapids, MI: Zondervan, 2001), 38.

5. Gary Chapman, *The Five Love Languages: The Secret to Love That Lasts* (Chicago: Northfield, 2010).

6. Robert M. Gray and David O. Moberg, *The Church and the Older Person* (Grand Rapids, MI: Eerdmans, 1962), 57.

7. James M. Houston and Michael Parker, *A Vision for the Aging Church: Renewing Ministry for and by Seniors* (Downers Grove, IL: IVP Academic, 2001), 72–90.

8. David P. Gallagher, *Senior Adult Ministry in the 21st Century: Step-by-Step Strategies for Reaching People Over 50* (Loveland, CO: Group, 2002), 13–25.

9. Gregory Waybright, "Local Church Ministry to and through Older Adults," in *Aging, Death and the Quest for Immortality*, ed. C. Ben Mitchell, Robert Orr, and Susan Saliday (Grand Rapids, MI: Eerdmans, 2004), 109.

10. M. W. Parker and G. Fuller, "Successful Aging," in *Finishing Strong* (Dallas: LifeWay, 2002), 63–70.

11. Dietrich Bonhoeffer, *Life Together: The Classic Exploration of Faith in Community*, trans. John Doberstein (San Francisco, Harper, 1954), 97.

12. Ibid., 99.

13. Ibid., 100.

14. Ibid., 103ff.

15. Ibid., 110ff.

16. For a fuller discussion of these issues see John Dunlop, *Finishing Well to the Glory of God: Strategies from a Christian Physician* (Wheaton, IL: Crossway, 2011), 41–45.

17. Frank E. Graeff, "Does Jesus Care?," 1901.

Chapter 5: Financial Wellness

1. "John D. Rockefeller," http://www.newworldencyclopedia.org/entry/John_D._Rockefeller (accessed July 17, 2012).
2. "Benjamin Franklin," http://www.iwise.com/Benjamin_Franklin (accessed July 17, 2012).
3. "Billy Graham," Gaiam Life, http://blog.gaiam.com/quotes/authors/billy-graham/5233 (accessed July 17, 2012).
4. "Jim Elliott," Wikipedia.org, http://en.wikipedia.org/wiki/Jim_Elliot (accessed July 17, 2012).
5. "Health, United States 2011," http://www.cdc.gov/nchs/data/hus/hus11.pdf#022 (accessed May 21, 2013).
6. Brian Kluth, *Experience God as Your Provider: Finding Financial Stability in Unstable Times* (Chicago: Moody, 2010), 88.

Chapter 6: Spiritual Wellness

1. Augustine, *Confessions*, http://www.goodreads.com/quotes/8308-thou-hast-made-us-for -thyself-o-lord-and-our (accessed May 20, 2013).
2. D. A. Carson, *For the Love of God: A Daily Companion for Discovering the Riches of God's Word*, 2 vols. (Wheaton IL: Crossway, 1999), 2:Apr. 23.

Chapter 7: Emotional Wellness

1. If you are not familiar with these delightful characters, you have missed an essential part of your education. Get hold of a Winnie-the-Pooh book, find a young child, read away, and enjoy.
2. David B. Biebel and Harold G. Koenig, *New Light on Depression: Help, Hope, and Answers for the Depressed and Those Who Love Them* (Grand Rapids MI: Zondervan, 2004), 90–91.
3. "Charles Spurgeon: Preaching through Adversity," Desiring God, http://www.desiring god.org/resource-library/biographies/charles-spurgeon-preaching-through-adversity (accessed May 21, 2013).
4. Chris R. Armstrong, "Martin Luther's Anfechtungen—His Own Dark Night of the Soul and How It Affected His Teaching and Ministry," http://gratefultothedead.wordpress .com/2011/08/24/martin-luthers-anfechtungen-his-own-dark-nights-of-the-soul-and -how-they-affected-his-teaching-and-ministry (accessed December 29, 2012).
5. Jonathan Edwards, *A Treatise Concerning Religious Affection* (West Roxbury, MA: B&R Samizdat Express), Kindle e-book, 15.
6. Johnson Oatman Jr., "Count Your Blessings," Timeless Truths Free Online, http://library .timelesstruths.org/music/Count_Your_Blessings/ (accessed January 28, 2013).
7. Stephen Sapp, *Full of Years: Aging and the Elderly in the Bible and Today* (Nashville: Abingdon, 1987), 141.
8. Jeremiah Burroughs, *The Rare Jewel of Christian Contentment* (Carlisle, PA: Banner of Truth, 1998), 13.

General Index

factors contributing to, 32; and God, 33, 46; medical care for, 42–43; and medications, 44–45; and preventative care, 43–44; and rest, 40; and surgery, 46–47; and unsafe behaviors, 42; and weight, 33
physician, choosing, 42–43
preventative care, 43–44

relationships; building, 88–96; categories of, 157; with the elderly, 141; with family, 95–96; with the Lord, 19, 23–24, 27, 43, 77, 86–87, 123–44, 135, 166; loss of, 96–98; social, 20, 77–99, 156; as two-way streets, 24; with the young, 160
resilience, 163–64
rest; and sleep, 40–41; and stress, 40
retirement, 82–82, 85, 89, 96, 101, 113–114, 116, 118

sanctification, 137
Sapp, Stephen (*Full of Years*), 161–62
sarcopenia, 35
self-pity, 148–49
Sell, Charles (Chick), 14
Senior Adult Ministry in the 21st Century (Gallagher), 92
serving the Lord, 45, 80, 87, 92, 153
shalom; definition of, 23; examples of, 23–25; and God, 23–25, 26
Shema, 23, 24, 27
sin; confessing, 94–95; and contentment, 165; curse of, 148; and difficulties, 20; and sanctification, 137; saved from, 26; turning from, 142; victory over, 136–37; and work, 89
Singh, Fauja (Turbaned Tornado), 18
social wellness; through church involvement, 90–95; through companionship, 17–18, 77; and family, 95–96; and friendships, 77–79, 94–95; and God, 78, 86–87; and living situation, 88–92; in loss, 96–98; and marriage, 80–84; during retirement, 89–90

spending, prudent, 114–15
spiritual wellness, 19, 20; and attitude, 143–44; beginning of, 123–27; and church involvement, 134; and fruit of the Spirit, 134–35; and God, 123–24, 125, 131 142; life transformation of, 133–34; planning for, 20–21; and repentance, 137; and serving, 138–43; and spiritual disciplines, 135–36; and spiritual growth, 128–31; through surrendering control, 126; and trust in God, 131–32
stewardship; of the body, 33, 36, 38, 44, 46, 149; and financial planning, 111–12, 114–15, 149; of the mind, 50
Sudden Infant Death Syndrome (SIDS), 141
surgery, 45–46

Tai Chi, 36
television viewing, 35, 41, 52, 86

unsafe behaviors, 42

Vision for the Aging Church, A (Houston and Parker), 91–92, 93

Waybright, Gregory (*Aging, Death and the Quest for Immortality*), 92
wealth, biblical advice for, 110–20
Weight Watchers, 37
wellness; areas of, 18; definition of, 18–19, 21–22, 47, 147; and faith in Christ, 11, 14; and God, 12, 13, 15, 20, 21, 22, 27; planning for, 20; and *shalom*, 23, 24; strategies for, 12, 13, 14, 15, 20
work, continuing, 89–90
worry; constructive, 149, 150; destructive, 150; and financial wellness, 102, 106, 108, 113, 120, 121, 165; and trust in God, 150, 151

Scripture Index

Also Available from John Dunlop, MD.

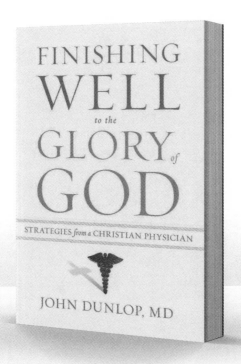

"Drawing from his years of experience as a physician who has shepherded countless patients through the 'valley of the shadow of death,' Dunlop provides pastoral wisdom and sound strategies. He gently addresses spiritual, emotional, psychological, financial, and physical needs. This book helps us plan our final decades, months, weeks, and hours with a God-centered attitude toward death and dying."

PAIGE CUNNINGHAM, *Executive Director, The Center for Bioethics and Human Dignity*

"Don't face your death or that of a loved one unprepared. *Finishing Well* is the most comprehensive, deeply Christian, and readable resource I know of its kind, and will prepare you and your loved ones to die well."

DAVID STEVENS, MD, *CEO, Christian Medical and Dental Association*

"The strategies Dunlop offers are clearly the result of years of experience in caring for persons in their twilight years. This book will be helpful for patients and families both before death and afterward."

ROBERT ORR, MD, *Professor of Medical Ethics, Loma Linda University, Center for Christian Bioethics*